HIGH-FIBER COOKING

A collection of delicious recipes to inspire you to a healthier
way of eating.

HIGH-FIBER COOKING

by

JANETTE MARSHALL

Illustrated by Ian Jones

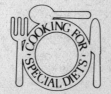

THORSONS PUBLISHERS LIMITED
New York

Thorsons Publishers Inc.
377 Park Avenue South
New York, New York 10016

First U.S. Edition 1984

LIBRARY OF CONGRESS CATALOGING IN PUBLICATION DATA

Marshall, Janette
  High-fiber cooking.
  Includes index.
  1. High-fiber diet—Recipes. I. Title.
RM237.6.M37 1984 641.5'637 83-24351
ISBN 0-7225-0818-2

Printed and bound in Great Britain by
Richard Clay (The Chaucer Press) Ltd., Bungay, Suffolk

Thorsons Publishers Inc. are distributed to the trade by
Inner Traditions International Ltd., New York

CONTENTS

ACKNOWLEDGEMENT

I should like to thank *Here's Health* magazine for allowing me to use some of the recipes devised for cookery articles in that magazine.

This book is dedicated to better health.

PART 1

1.

WHY ALL THE FUSS ABOUT FIBER?

For many thousands of years man lived on natural foods. He grew cereals and ground them with stones to make rough breads and porridges and he gathered root vegetables, fruits and berries. His eating pattern was high in dietary fiber. It is only very recently (in evolutionary terms) that he has started to take the fiber out of his food. Why . . .?

Fiber is removed to refine foods. The best example is the milling of flour. When white flour is produced the bran (the outer coating of the wheat grain) is removed along with the wheat germ. Essential nutrients like B vitamins and vitamin E are also lost in order to produce a more sophisticated, white product.

The white flour is more concentrated than its unrefined counterpart, whole wheat flour. For the same volume of flour you are getting more starch at the expense of other nutrients and fiber. White flour is an example of a refined carbohydrate (starch food) and whole wheat flour is an unrefined carbohydrate.

Another example of a refined carbohydrate is sugar. By removing all the fiber and nutrients from a large sugar beet one teaspoon of white sugar is produced — an even more concentrated food than white flour. White sugar is pure carbohydrate with no protein, vitamins, minerals or fat; it is 100 per cent carbohydrate offering only calories.

On the face of it refining food would seem to be a good idea. After all, it strips the food to a more concentrated form of carbohydrate, and because these foods are eaten for energy it will give us that energy quicker without having to digest a lot of other ingredients as well.

It would *seem* to have another advantage too. Removing fiber and concentrating foods makes them sweeter, and man has a sweet tooth. In fact the experience of the last 150 years, since man started refining these carbohydrate foods on a large scale, has shown them *not* to have any advantages. The opposite has happened with definite ill effects on health.

What is Fiber?

Fiber is the substance that makes up the cell walls of plants. If you imagine a cell to be like a cardboard box, the fiber is the equivalent of the sides of the box. Pile several boxes on top of each other and you have a simplified illustration of the way the fiber in plant cell walls enables the plant to stay upright.

Animal cells do not contain fiber, but that doesn't mean animals are always falling over! Humans and animals are kept upright by their skeleton. Muscles are attached to the bones to move the body about. This basic difference is important because it highlights the fact that fiber is only available in plant foods. Meat, fish and dairy products are devoid of fiber.

Not all plants contain the same amount or type of fiber. Trees, for example, have "high fiber" trunks and branches, but they are not much use to man from a culinary point of view (apart from providing the table from which to eat).

The types of plants that are high in fiber often give themselves away by their texture. Legumes (dried beans, peas and lentils) are good sources and so are cereals (wheat, oats, barley, rice and rye) and dried fruits (dates, prunes, figs, apricots). Fresh vegetables and fruits (particularly blackberries, raspberries and other fruits with many tiny seeds) are also naturally high in fiber.

What Does Fiber Do?

Cereal fiber, the bran from wheat, oats and other grains, is best known as a remedy for constipation. Coarse bran seems to be more effective than fine bran because it can absorb more water and so form a soft bulk that will speed evacuation of waste from the body. How it works is dealt with more fully under the headings Constipation (page 19) and Diverticulitis (page 21).

Fruit fiber is in the form of pectin (the substance that makes jams and jellies jell) which dissolves in water but is resistant to digestive enzymes. This jelling effect softens stools and is protective against some toxins (see Cancer of the Colon, page 24).

Lignin is another type of fiber that forms as plants mature. Soft young fruit and vegetables contain little; it is more likely to be found in the outer leaves of cabbages and the woody core of carrots. Lignin is also found in cereals. It is the type of dietary fiber that binds with bile salts and takes them quickly from the body (see Gallstones, page 23).

2.

WHAT HAPPENS WHEN YOU EAT TOO MUCH LOW-FIBER FOOD?

Obesity

When fiber is removed from food it makes it a lot easier to eat. Take, for example, that teaspoon of sugar. If we had to eat the sugar beet in its natural state it would take a lot longer than a quick dip into the sugar bowl and a quick stir of the tea or coffee. All the calories of that large vegetable (or sugar cane) have been concentrated to fit neatly into a teaspoon.

Perhaps you are saying, "Who eats sugar beet anyway?" If you are, try applying the example to other foods. White flour for example will be made into bread, or cakes and pastries. Consider how many slices of white bread it takes to make you feel "full-up". Then compare that with how much whole wheat bread is needed for the same job. If you are not feeling hungry here is the answer. It takes more white bread, and that means more calories and fewer vitamins and minerals and less fiber. Why?

Whole wheat bread is made from flour that is just milled wheat grains. None of the bran or wheat germ is removed and none of the nutrients are lost. It is the "wholeness" of wholewheat bread and the natural dietary fiber that fills you up. Because it is an unrefined and unconcentrated food it has more bulk and less calories. Therefore it fills you up and leaves you slimmer.

When the fiber has been removed from food the body can use the energy quicker. Fiber has a slowing effect on digestion; without this slowing effect the food is converted into energy very soon after it is eaten. It is then taken into the bloodstream causing a sudden rise in the amount of sugar in the blood. The blood takes the sugar to the cells where the energy is burned up, and you feel hungry again in a short time. There's no surer pattern of eating to lead to a weight problem. Especially as the slump in energy after a refined/sugary meal leads to that empty feeling and craving for something sweet, like chocolate, for more "instant" energy.

Fiber for Slimming

Switching to fiber-rich foods can solve this food-craving problem for the overweight. By choosing high-fiber foods you will be getting:

★ less concentrated forms of calories;

★ food that takes longer to digest leaving you feeling full for longer;

★ food that needs chewing which takes longer to eat and helps you feel that you have "eaten";

★ food that contains essential vitamins and minerals, often missing from non-wholefood slimming diets that restrict the variety of foods normally containing these nutrients;

★ better health by avoiding constipation often associated with dieting;

★ more chance of losing weight because when fiber is present during digestion a larger proportion of calories remain undigested.

Diabetes

Diabetes occurs when there is a lack of effective insulin. Insulin is a hormone produced in the pancreas. It is responsible for dealing with sugar once it has been absorbed into the blood from the intestine. During digestion carbohydrates are broken down into their constituent sugars which fuel the body with energy, and it is the job of insulin to make this energy available to the body. Without enough insulin, sugar will build up in the blood, starving the body of energy. Because the sugar cannot be used it will be excreted in the urine.

Diabetes usually occurs either in children (when it is often the result of an inherited disposition) or, more commonly, in middle-age when it is called maturity-onset diabetes. The latter type of diabetes can be helped by diet, often obviating recourse to insulin.

In maturity-onset diabetes the body produces insulin, but it is ineffective. This type of diabetes is usually accompanied by a weight problem and it can sometimes be controlled simply by regaining normal weight. As normal weight is regained the body loses its resistance to its own insulin.

If the problem is solved, then the switch in diet to eating more unrefined foods (often called wholefoods because they are the whole foods in their natural state) should be maintained to prevent further weight gain (see Fiber for Slimming, page 15). A wholefood, high-fiber eating pattern will also help some diabetics keep their blood sugar levels stable without using insulin. This can be illustrated by a look at the way insulin works in the body.

As we have seen, carbohydrates are broken down into their constituent sugars during digestion and pass from the intestine into the blood. When they enter the bloodstream insulin is produced because it is needed in order for the sugar to be absorbed. A sugary meal or snack leads to a sudden influx of blood sugar which the body has to quickly respond to by producing insulin. The sudden demand often leads to overproduction which clears the bloodstream efficiently but results in an equally quick slump in blood sugar. Eating meals of unrefined carbohydrates produces a steadier stream of sugar which does not make sudden demands on insulin production or lead to overproduction.

Long-term use of refined carbohydrates, especially very concentrated forms like sugary foods and sweets, will make unreasonable demands on the insulin-producing pancreas and makes susceptibility to diabetes more likely.

Low Blood Sugar
This condition can be another result of eating too many low-fiber foods, and it is becoming increasingly common. The rapid digestion of low-fiber foods causes a sudden influx of sugar to the blood which makes sudden demands on insulin-producing glands (see Diabetes, page 15). Often blood sugar levels are depressed before insulin

production returns to normal and a chemical state of diabetes can be caused, with the person often feeling dizzy.

If the insulin keeps on being produced it will cause the body to dig into its fat stores to convert fat quickly into glucose for the insulin to work on, and this will raise the level of fat in the bloodstream. This excess of fat and sugar can lead to arteriosclerosis (see Coronary Heart Disease, below).

Again, fiber-rich foods can come to the rescue by providing a steady stream of fuel for the body that does not make undue demands on insulin production.

Coronary Heart Disease

Both the overweight and diabetics are more likely to develop heart disease. Recent research has suggested that prevention of heart disease may be helped with a high-fiber diet.

Coronary heart disease is a disease of the arteries that supply blood to the heart muscle. The diseased arteries can become coated with deposits that narrow the passages through which the blood flows. In this way they can prevent the heart receiving all the blood (and thus oxygen) it needs to work properly. The arteries may even silt up completely, or a blood clot may lodge in a narrowed artery preventing blood reaching the heart muscle. If the blood supply to the heart is cut off completely a heart attack happens. In less serious cases partial restriction of blood supply causes heart failure.

Heart disease, like diabetics, is prevalent in countries where a diet of unrefined carbohydrates (a typical Western diet) is eaten. This type of diet is also high in fats, especially animal fats. There are other risk factors in coronary heart disease, including smoking, obesity, lack of exercise, raised blood pressure, too much sugary food, excess salt, and diabetes.

Most research has concentrated on the effects of fats, especially animal fats, in heart disease, but researchers have also noticed how low-fiber diets often accompany coronary heart disease. A lot of attention has been paid to the role of cholesterol because it is a major component of the arterial plaque that narrows artery walls. So preventive coronary heart disease measures have included ways of cutting the amount of cholesterol circulating in the blood so that less can be deposited on arterial walls.

Fiber has been shown to have an important part to play in lowering the amount of cholesterol in circulation. Oats have been shown to be very effective because their fiber binds with the type of fats that are deposited as arterial plaque and removes them from the body, leaving the type of fats that are essential for health in circulation.

There is also the general health benefit that the more unrefined carbohydrates you eat, the less room there is in the diet for refined foods that are high in fat and refined sugar which are both implicated in coronary heart disease.

Research is also examining the role of fiber in preventing the formation of blood clots. Heart attacks can occur when blood clots form in arteries, and clots happen more frequently in Western people than African and other Third World people. Studies on rural Africans have shown their body chemistry can break up clots quicker than Western body chemistry.

3.

THE OTHER EFFECTS OF LOW-FIBER FOODS

Constipation

This must be one of the commonest complaints in Western civilization. It cost the National Health Service in Britain £7,310,000 ($11,000,000) in 1981 for laxative prescriptions. Now more and more doctors are advising their patients to increase the fiber in their diet by taking bran as the simplest solution.

Adding bran to a diet of refined carbohydrates will not solve anything. It will only mask symptoms caused by fiberless foods.

Advice given for treating constipation relies to a great extent on the definition of constipation. Some doctors still believe that a regular and normal evacuation of the bowel once every five days is not constipation if that is "normal" for a particular person. However, informed opinion does not now regard that as "normal".

Research by surgeon Mr Dennis Burkitt, a pioneer of the modern appreciation of the importance of fiber in the diet, has compared bowel movements of African people living on an unrefined, natural diet with bowel movements of those eating a Western refined diet. His studies showed that the frequency and volume of the bowel movements of the two groups differed widely. Those on a more fibrous diet would experience one or two bowel motions daily, evacuating up to and over ½ kilo of feces. The Western diet produced daily bowel motions of a few ounces. He also noticed important differences in the time taken for food to pass through the body and differences in consistency of the waste matter.

Some people may find it obsessive and cranky to consider such things, but Mr Burkitt's findings and the findings of others, have a great bearing on health. They also highlight the dangers of a low-fiber diet and the high price to be paid in terms of health for habitual reliance on laxatives.

Habitual use of laxatives results in a bowel that is unable to function without this stimulation. In such cases a person will regard as "normal" the daily large volume of fluid stool that has been induced. However this is a dangerous situation and deprives the body of valuable salts which may result in major surgery to a damaged colon.

Acceptance of a small bowel motion once or twice a week is also potentially dangerous. Such bowel movements are probably "normal" in people eating a diet of refined carbohydrates, but like the refined diet they are not natural.

A lot of wrongful application of laxatives has arisen because of the misunderstanding of the word constipation. It really refers to the difficulty in passing hard stools and not to the length of time between bowel movements. The physical straining involved in evacuating hard stools can lead to more serious diseases and this is one reason why constipation should be avoided. Another reason is that the longer waste products of digestion remain in the digestive tract the greater the risk of reabsorbing dangerous toxins.

The transit time of food through the body was measured by Mr Burkitt, who found that an African diet of high-fiber natural foods passed through the system in about 1½ days. The transit time of a Western diet was between three days in a healthy young person and two weeks in an elderly person. The amount of fiber in the diet bore a direct correlation to the transit time.

As food passes through the gut the body absorbs water from it. The drier the food becomes the harder and more compacted it becomes, which makes it more difficult for the muscle in the gut to squeeze it along. The action of fiber in food is like a sponge. It soaks up water and keeps the food mass soft. As it soaks up the water it enlarges and gives the waste a soft bulk that is easier for the muscles to move. It therefore stays in the gut for a shorter time, which has several advantages:

● it prevents physical straining to pass hard stools and therefore *removes constipation;*

● it reduces the time undigested waste material spends in contact with the intestine (see Cancer of the Colon, page 24), so it *protects against toxic material.*

Hemorrhoids, Varicose Veins and Hiatus Hernia

These three conditions are common among people eating a typical refined diet, and they have been grouped together because they can be the direct result of constipation.

For a long time hemorrhoids were thought to be anal varicose veins, but now it is thought they are a prolapse of part of the anal region which is full of blood vessels. The prolapse is caused by straining during constipation.

Veins are the vessels that return the blood to the heart after the oxygen has been delivered to body cells via the arteries. The veins contain valves to stop the blood flowing backwards against the flow of gravity, which it is likely to do in regions such as the legs. During abdominal straining such as constipation the blood is forced to flow back down the legs causing the valves to stretch. Eventually they will not be able to function properly and varicose veins will develop. An hereditory disposition can make some people more susceptible to varicose veins.

Hiatus hernias are another direct result of straining during constipation. They are prevalent in middle-aged people who eat a low-fiber diet. The hernia results when pressure in the abdomen builds up (during straining at stool) and the top of the stomach is forced through the hole in the diaphragm through which the digestive tract passes.

Diverticulitis

This disease, characterized by pockets or pouches in the wall of the colon, is another modern health problem that has developed along with the increased consumption of refined foods. It began to appear in medical textbooks after the 1920s and was, by 1960, the most common disease of the colon in the West. More than one third of people are thought to have diverticula by the time they are forty.

At first it was thought that diverticula were caused by constipation, but further investigation has shown the cause to be more likely a build-up of pressure in the colon.

Propelling a soft fecal mass along the colon produces regular waves of pressure, but moving a small, hard mass means that the colon walls have to contract further with greater force which causes areas of pressure to occur in the gaps between the hard fecal matter. These miniature pressure chambers cause small "blow-outs", or hernias, in the colon wall producing pockets (diverticula) in the same way as an inner tube bulges through the outer wall of a tire.

When diverticulitis was first recognized patients were treated with bland, fiber-depleted diets because it was thought that "roughage" would aggravate the gut. More modern research has shown that a high-fiber diet is more beneficial. It cannot cure diverticulitis because the condition is not reversible, but it can remove the original problem (hard fecal matter) and prevent further occurrences. It can also make life more comfortable by eliminating constipation. Dyspeptic pains and localized colic pains have also been reduced among some patients who have tried a high-fiber diet.

Duodenal Ulcers

Traditional treatment for ulcers has been a bland diet free from roughage; this has also been turned on its head by recent discoveries of the role of fiber in the diet.

A Norwegian study compared the health of seventy-three recently healed duodenal ulcer patients who ate either a high-fiber diet based on unrefined carbohydrates or a low-fiber diet devoid of these foods. The high-fiber group experienced only forty-five per cent relapses compared with eighty per cent relapses in the low-fiber group.

The high-fiber diet is thought to benefit ulcer patients by stopping the liquids which normalize acidity in the stomach from leaving the area before their work is finished — which they have a tendency to do when there is no fiber in the food to absorb them and keep them in the stomach.

Appendicitis

This is a health problem rarely found among people of Africa and the Third World, but like heart disease it is something that such people develop when they move to urbanized environments with Western diet. It is a disease with substantial evidence to show that a high-fiber diet, and whole wheat bread consumption in particular, lessens the incidence.

The number of cases of appendicitis in England and Wales dropped between 1971 and 1975, and reports in the British medical press have shown the decrease to be concurrent with an increase in the consumption of whole wheat bread, fresh fruit and vegetables.

Appendicitis occurs when the appendix, a blind-ended tube of about two inches (5cm) in length found at the beginning of the large intestine, becomes blocked and subsequently infected. The blockage is usually caused by a small lump of hard feces, typically the type of feces of a low-fiber diet. If the feces are soft there is less likelihood of an appendix blockage and infection occurring.

Gallstones

Gallstones are formed in the bile duct leading from the gall bladder to the intestine. Like cancer of the colon, bile salts are involved in the development of this disease. After meals, the gall bladder secretes bile which contains substances necessary to digest fatty foods. Bile is made from cholesterol, and bile salts and stones are formed when there is too much cholesterol and not enough of one of the bile salts that prevents the cholesterol crystallizing into gallstones.

Increasing the amount of fiber in the diet has been shown to result in production of bile that contains less cholesterol. It also seems to encourage bile that is more likely to keep the cholesterol in solution and therefore not let it crystallize into stones. Fiber also seems to bind and excrete undesirable bile salts and prevents them from getting back into the system. It can also bind cholesterol during digestion and prevent it being absorbed; this is not only good news for gallstone sufferers but for dieters and heart disease sufferers.

High Blood Pressure

This is one of the risk factors in some types of heart disease and is usually found among middle-aged and older people, although some pregnant women also experience high blood pressure.

Once again this is a disease predominant in Westernized people and rarely found in people eating a primitive, unrefined diet. Among Western people vegetarians have been shown to suffer less from high blood pressure than their meat-eating peers; the vegetarian diet is typically high-fiber and low-fat.

Experiments at Southampton University have shown that students with a high-fiber intake had lower blood pressure than those with a low-fiber intake. When those on a high-fiber diet switched to a low-fiber intake their blood pressure showed marked increases within four weeks. The reverse was also true; increasing fiber intake reduced blood pressure. (The same effect was seen when switching from unsaturated fats to saturated fats; the former having a beneficial effect on blood pressure.) Reducing salt intake also helps lower high blood pressure.

Not only were cholesterol levels lower in those on a high-fiber diet but perhaps more importantly fiber was also able to alter the blood chemistry in a beneficial way. High density lipo-protein (HDL), which is thought to be protective against heart disease, was increased in high-fiber eaters and low density lipo-protein, thought to be harmful, was lowered. Oat fiber is now known to be especially effective in this area.

As well as these influences on blood pressure it is likely that fiber has an influence on hormones that cause high blood pressure. Fiber has already been seen to influence production of the hormone insulin (see Diabetes, page 15).

The slimming effect (see Obesity, page 14) of fiber is also of benefit to high blood pressure sufferers who are often overweight.

Cancer of the Colon

Like other diseases of the digestive tract, cancer of the colon has been related to diet. Cancer of the gut usually occurs in the colon or rectum where it is thought that bacteria cause chemical changes in the food being digested which produce carcinogens (cancer-inducing substances).

The type of diet that has been shown to predispose towards gut cancers is one that is low in unrefined cereals and high in animal fats. Low incidence (or absence) of colon cancer in people of Africa and

Asia, who eat diets low in animal fat and high in unrefined cereals, has meant that their diet is seen as protective against such cancers.

Fats increase the amount of bile salts in the colon which the bacteria may convert into carcinogens. A high-fiber diet usually results in less fat being eaten because hunger can be satiated without recourse to fatty foods and so the amount of potentially harmful bile salts is reduced.

Fiber also provides bulking material that absorbs water which dilutes any carcinogens present. It also moves the waste material and harmful substances through the body quicker so they spend less time in contact with the walls of the intestine through which they may otherwise be reabsorbed into the blood.

Fiber not only removes carcinogens from the body but it also seems to absorb other poisonous substances in its mass and prevents them being reabsorbed.

Breast Cancer

Breast cancer has been linked with diet in various ways, one of which involves fiber as a preventive. Recent medical research has come round to the long-held naturopathic opinion that women's breasts take up toxic waste products that have been reabsorbed into the bloodstream from waste material that lingers in the large intestine.

Associations have been noted between constipation and lumpy breasts, chronic cystic disease and cancer. Cystic disease has been seen to improve when constipation is relieved. The way to avoid constipation is, as has been seen, to eat a wholefood, high-fiber diet.

Lumpy breasts can also be caused by changes in hormone balance which are sometimes brought about through changes in the levels of fat in the diet. (The effects of fiber on fat have been seen in Gallstones, Heart Disease, High Blood Pressure.)

Although the interplay of fiber, gut bacteria and absorption of carcinogenic toxins from waste in the gut needs fuller investigation, research has so far indicated that vegetarian women on a high-fiber diet are afforded some protection against breast cancer by their diet. This is thought to be because fiber influences the production of beneficial estrogen hormones (usually found in higher levels in vegetarian women) which are protective. Women with severe mastalgia and breast swelling are also known to find relief on macrobiotic and high-fiber diets. The role of vitamin A, found in high-fiber vegetables like carrots and dark green vegetables, may also be linked to vegetarians' protection.

Lung Cancer

A ten-year study in Holland which scrutinized the diet and medical histories of 1000 middle-aged men confirmed that low-fiber intake increases the risks of heart disease and other diseases associated with low-fiber intake. It also highlighted the less well-known link of low-fiber diet and deaths from cancer. Surprisingly lung cancer occurred significantly more in the low-fiber intake group where the men's diets lacked beta-carotene found in carrots and dark green vegetables (both of which are high-fiber vegetables).

Teeth and Gums

Teeth and gums, as well as general health, will benefit from a high-fiber wholefood diet. The fresh fruit and vegetables, whole wheat bread, grains and legumes will mean less room for sticky cakes, pastries, cookies and sweets. Less sugar to cling around the teeth. The chewing and crunching of wholefoods will keep the mouth clean and fresh and help ensure only the right kind of bacteria take up residence.

4.

TAKING PREVENTIVE ACTION

How to Get More Fiber

Taking the easy way out and reaching for a packet of bran to sprinkle on food, or switching to a sugary bran breakfast cereal is not the best way to get more fiber. Adding bran to a diet based on refined foods such as white bread, white flour, cakes and pastries and high in meat and dairy products is not the way to avoid constipation and its associated health problems.

Changing to a wholefood diet is the best way to get more fiber.

For one thing bran on its own is not as effective in reducing blood cholesterol levels as eating the whole grain as near to its natural state as possible. Bran may be an effective first aid measure but it is as "unnatural" as the ingredients of a refined diet in which foods have been removed from their natural state by food processing.

Adding large amounts of bran may even have temporary ill effects. Critics of whole wheat bread proponents have often said that the phytic acid found in bran can damage health by blocking absorption of minerals like calcium and zinc by binding them into forms that the body cannot use. However, experiments have shown that detrimental effects of phytic acid in whole wheat bread are only temporary; after about six weeks the body adjusts and the calcium balance is restored to normal.

Overdoing the addition of bran will also result in larger than normal stools which may cause discomfort and fissures (small anal tears) and may also result in diarrhea and irregular bowel habits.

The best way to increase fiber is to switch to natural, unprocessed foods which will provide a steady stream of energy and which come complete with natural amounts of fiber.

Foods to Choose for Fiber

Whole wheat bread, crispbreads.

Whole wheat flour, soy flour, rye flour.

Oats, as oatcakes and as a base for homemade, no-added-sugar muesli.

Whole wheat pastry; try adding oats and oatmeal sometimes for a change.

Brown rice, and other grains like millet, barley, whole wheat berries.

Whole wheat pasta.

Legumes such as dried beans, peas, lentils — even baked beans.

Fresh fruit, washed but unpeeled.

Fresh vegetables, washed but unpeeled where possible, or cooked in their jackets like baked potatoes or sweet potatoes. Peas and beans are also high in fiber and when choosing lettuce choose a crispy variety which has more fiber than floppy leaved types. Use outer leaves.

Dried fruits like apricots, prunes, dates, coconut, raisins, golden seedless raisins, currants, peaches, pears etc.

Nuts and seeds.

Non-Fiber Foods in the Wholefood Diet

Free-range eggs.

Natural yogurt.

No-added-sugar jams and marmalades.

Fish, for essential fatty acids.

Herb teas, mineral water and fruit and vegetable juices (in moderation) in place of stimulants like tea and coffee.

Decaffeinated coffee.

Dry white wine and hard cider (in moderation, 1½ glasses a day).

Cold-pressed vegetable oils. Use sunflower, safflower and olive oil for cold uses and the more stable corn oil and olive oil for cooking.

Small amounts of natural Cheddar-type cheeses.

Low-fat soft white curd, cream and other white cheeses.

Polyunsaturated soft vegetable margarines or unsalted butter.

Margarines have the advantage of being polyunsaturated (if you choose those varieties) but some people prefer the flavor of butter and the fact that it is less "processed" than margarine. Mixtures of the two can be used.

Organically Grown
Ask for organically grown vegetables and try to find a local supplier (or grow your own) because they are grown without the use of poisonous chemical fertilizers, sprays, pesticides, etc.

Flatulence
This problem often puts people off wholefoods when they try them. Remember that it won't last forever. Once your body is accustomed to its new diet this problem will disappear.

Natural yogurt may help alleviate some flatulence problems, but it is best to wean yourself gently onto wholefoods. First cut down on sugar and introduce whole wheat flour in place of white flour and whole wheat bread in place of white bread. Half and half flour mixtures could be used at first, gradually phasing out the white. Then try whole wheat pasta and introduce more fresh fruit and vegetables before trying dried beans, peas and lentils.

How Much Fiber to Aim For
Trying to add up the amount of fiber you are eating each day is no fun. Unless you like measuring each mouthful against tables and charts or have a photographic memory for figures it will be very boring and not an enjoyable approach to food. *It makes more sense to apply the principles of wholefood eating and forget about fiber. A wholefood diet will provide it naturally without you having to think about it.*

There is no "official" recommended daily allowance of fiber; if there was it would probably be an underestimate, but Burkitt (see Constipation, page 19) and others have found that as little as half to one ounce (15-25g) is eaten daily in the Western diet compared with one and a half to two ounces daily (40-60g) in undeveloped countries. Not a lot of difference, but it makes all the difference. Generally accepted figures seem to point to about 1½ oz (30-35g) a day as a good level. It is not recommended to exceed 2 oz (50g) a day.

A recent Dutch study on 1000 middle-aged men set the magic

protective figure at 37 grams a day. Researchers studied the diet and medical histories of the men for ten years. They revealed that mortality was four times higher in the low-fiber eaters. The men who died from low-fiber related diseases (see Lung Cancer, page 26) had an average intake of 27 grams a day with survivors averaging 31 grams, mostly from whole wheat bread, vegetables and vegetable protein. Those who did not survive the study also ate more animal foods than the survivors.

Celiacs

Celiacs have an intolerance to gluten, the protein content of wheat, barley, rye and oats. They must therefore derive their fiber from other sources such as brown rice, whole millet, whole corn, chickpea flour (garbanzo flour), chickpeas (garbanzo beans), cornmeal, lentils, beans, fresh and dried fruits, nuts, fresh vegetables.

Typical Day's High-Fiber Eating

Choose from the following suggestions.

Breakfast

Whole wheat toast with a scrape of unsalted butter or polyunsaturated margarine or low-fat soft white cheese.

No-added-sugar jams, marmalades, honey, barley malt.

Home-made muesli including oats, barley flakes, millet, sunflower seeds, sesame or pumpkin seeds, dried fruits, nuts, with natural yogurt, fruit juice or mineral water.

Porridge, with oat flakes, rolled oats or oatmeal.

Dried or fresh fruits.

Natural yogurt.

Eggs (free-range), boiled or scrambled (without fat or salt).

Baked beans.

Mushrooms, sweat in non-stick pan covered with lid to avoid addition of milk.

Milk, better without, but if using choose goat's milk or skimmed milk, raw milk is even better.

Mineral water.

Fresh fruit juice.

Herb tea.
Decaffeinated coffee.

Lunch
Whole wheat sandwiches.
Any salad vegetables.
Cottage or other low-fat cheese.
Open sandwiches of rye or pumpernickel bread.
Pizza.
Cold pasta, from the night before.
Rice, from the night before, with vegetables.
Beans, peas or lentils, from night before, with salad vegetables.
Whole wheat quiches.
Savory scones.
Muesli.
Whole wheat bread and taramasalata or hummus.

All these lunches can be eaten at home or taken as a packed lunch to work. They are also interchangeable with the Evening Meal if the main meal is eaten midday.

Evening Meal
Soups, using pasta, vegetables, legumes.
Salads, raw or just-blanched vegetables.
Fish, grilled or poached.
Poultry or game with skin removed; grilled, braised or casseroled.
Baked and stuffed potatoes.
Quiches and salads.
Bean dishes like chili con carne (use more beans than meat to increase fiber and cut fat consumption).
Rice dishes, paella, risotto, curry, stuffed vegetables.
Vegetable ratatouille, stir-fry, stews.
Whole wheat pasta, lasagne, spaghetti, tagliatelli, etc.
Whole wheat pot pies.
Stuffed whole wheat pancakes.

For recipes based on these ideas see recipe section.

Desserts
Natural yogurt, on its own, with honey or with fresh fruit.
Fresh fruit salads or platters.
Dried fruit compotes, mousses, fools, crumbles, tarts.
Pancakes with lemon juice and honey or fruit purées.
Cheesecakes made with cottage cheese, yogurt and fruit purées.
Stuffed fruit such as pears, apples.
Grilled bananas, grapefruit, oranges.

Snacks
Spiced teabreads and other yeast bread, in place of sweet cakes.
Whole wheat or oat crackers.
Fresh fruit.
Dried fruit.
Nuts.
Oatcakes.
Yogurts.
Whole wheat sandwiches.
Open crispbread sandwiches.
Pitta bread and salad.
Salads.
Soups.
Baked beans.
Baked potatoes.

5.
MENU SUGGESTIONS

Here are some menu suggestions that, taken together with the suggestions for breakfast and lunch, will ensure a healthy intake of fiber between 33 and 50 grams a day. Most importantly they are completely natural foods, high in fiber and they do not rely on the unnatural addition of bran. Each ingredient is in its natural state.

The dishes are interchangeable with others in the recipe section. Each recipe is marked with its fiber content per portion so it is possible for you to work out easily menus of your own choice that will add up to your daily fiber requirement.

Spring

Breakfast

Two whole wheat croissants   Two whole wheat croissants

Lunch

Four oatcakes with low-fat   Brown rice ring
  soft white cheese spread

Main Meal

Date and walnut salad   Fruit cocktail

★   ★

Tomato and olive pizza
with
Green bean and cashew salad

Broad bean minestrone
with
side salad of your choice

★

★

Hot fruit compote

Apricot and coconut crumble

Summer

Breakfast

Two breakfast buns

Two breakfast buns

Lunch

Pitta bread and salad

Niçoise pasta

Main Meal

Onion tart

Garden pea soup

★

★

Chickpea and marrow hotpot

Avocado and Brazil pancakes

★

★

Apricot rice

Gooseberry cheesecake

Autumn

Breakfast

Fruity porridge

Fruity porridge

Lunch

Baked cabbage

Leek and potato quiche

Main Meal

Watercress soup	Melon salad
★	★
Moussaka with side salad	Topped vegetables with Parsnip cheese
★	★
Jack Horner crumble	Peach galette

Winter

Breakfast

Coconut muesli	Coconut muesli

Lunch

Lentil soup	Chili baked potato

Main Meal

Persimmon cocktail	Celeriac soup
★	★
Dolmas	Groundnut stew with mangos and bananas
★	★
Prune jellies	Apricot gateau

Cooking Utensils

Aluminum saucepans have been the subject of suspicion for several years, mainly because they react with food. This can be seen when cooking acid foods, like fruit, in an aluminum pan. After cooking the pan is much shinier due to its reaction with the acid which may have made some aluminum come off into the food in minute amounts. These infinitesimal amounts may build up in the body over the years. Aluminum is not an "essential nutrient" for the body and it may even be harmful. For this reason it is best to choose stainless steel pans that do not react with food. Glassware, ceramic material and cast iron or enamelled cookware can also be used.

Meat and "Complete" Protein

This cookbook has not consciously set out to exclude meat, but because meat is devoid of fiber and high in saturated fats it does not make a useful contribution to a book that aims to outline practical ways to healthier eating.

Many of the vegetable dishes may be served with meat and they will usefully boost the fiber content of such a meal.

Fish is preferred to meat because it is an excellent source of protein and its fat is unsaturated. It also provides essential fatty acids that are beneficial to health.

The recipes in this book provide protein from vegetable sources because these are also sources of fiber. Vegetable proteins are not the "complete" proteins that meat, fish and dairy proteins are; they contain only a few of the essential building blocks needed by the body to make its own protein. However, by mixing proteins from vegetable sources "complete" proteins can be formed by the body.

To achieve complete proteins make sure the meal contains one of the following three combinations:

- grains (cereal, pasta, rice, etc.) with legumes (beans, peas or lentils);
- grains and milk products;
- seeds (sesame, sunflower, pumpkin) and legumes.

PART 2
THE RECIPES
6.
BREAKFASTS

COCONUT MUESLI
Serves 4.
5g fiber/250 calories per portion.

⅓ cup rolled oats
2 tablespoons wheat flakes
1 tablespoon sunflower seeds
1 tablespoon raisins
1 tablespoon slivered almonds
1 tablespoon ground coconut
1 tablespoon wheat germ

1. Mix all ingredients together very thoroughly to ensure fair shares of the nuts and raisins!

2. Place portions of muesli in breakfast bowls and soak overnight, in either fruit juice, such as apple juice, or mineral water. Natural yogurt or cultured buttermilk may also be used.

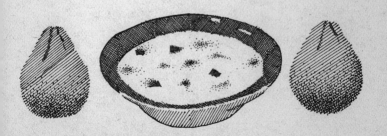

SIMPLE MUESLI
Serves 2.
3g fiber/300 calories per portion.

1/2 cup rolled oats
1 tablespoon raisins
1 tablespoon sunflower seeds
Apple juice or mineral water
3 or 4 hazelnuts
1 eating apple

1. Mix together the oats, raisins and sunflower seeds. Soak overnight in apple juice or water in the fridge.

2. Next morning chop the hazelnuts and grate the cored but unpeeled apple. Stir these into the muesli.

3. Add more juice or water or, if preferred, top with natural yogurt before serving.

BREAKFAST BUNS
Makes about 16.
3g fiber/110 calories each.

1 1/2 cups whole wheat flour
2 teaspoons baking powder
1/2 cup bran
1/4 cup polyunsaturated margarine
2 tablespoons clear honey
2/3 cup apple juice
2/3 cup raisins
3/4 cup chopped English walnuts
1 cooking apple, grated

1. Sieve the flour and baking powder into a bowl. Stir in the bran.

2. Place the margarine, honey and apple juice in a saucepan over gentle heat and melt.

3. Stir the raisins, walnuts and apple into the dry ingredients.

4. Pour over the melted ingredients and mix thoroughly. The mixture will be quite moist.

5. Place 1 tablespoonful of mixture into lightly oiled small muffin tins or paper cases.

6. Bake at 375°F for 25 minutes.

FRUITY PORRIDGE
Serves 4.
4½g fiber/240 calories per portion.

1½ cups rolled oats
½ cup wheat germ
⅓ cup raisins
Water
2 eating apples

1. Place the oats, wheat germ and raisins in a saucepan.

2. Add water and place over low heat. Bring to simmering point, stirring continuously to prevent sticking. The amount of water needed will depend on the absorbency of the oats and the texture at which porridge is preferred. Between 1⅓ and 2 cups will probably be enough.

3. Core, but do not peel the apples, and grate them into the porridge just before serving.

WHOLE WHEAT CROISSANTS
Makes 24.
2½g fiber/70 calories each.

2½ tablespoons fresh yeast, or 1 tablespoon dried yeast
1 vitamin C tablet
1 cup warm water
1 cup evaporated milk
¼ cup unsalted butter, melted
6 cups whole wheat flour
1 teaspoon sea salt (optional)
¾ cup unsalted butter
Milk to glaze

1. Crumble the yeast and crushed vitamin C tablet into the warm water.

2. Add the evaporated milk and stir well.

3. Melt the smaller amount of butter in saucepan. Remove from heat.

4. Sieve the flour and salt (if used) into a bowl.

5. Rub the larger amount of butter into the flour until it resembles breadcrumbs.

6. Make a well in center of the flour and pour in the yeast mixture and melted butter and mix thoroughly.

7. Turn onto a lightly floured surface and knead for 5 minutes. Return to bowl, cover and leave to rest for 10 minutes.

8. Turn ⅓ dough onto a lightly floured surface and roll into a circle with dough about ¼ in. thick.

9. Using a sharp knife cut the dough into eight segments. Working from the outside, roll each triangular segment into the middle to form a croissant roll. Bend into a crescent moon shape and place on lightly oiled baking tray. Cover and leave to double in size.

10. Repeat with other ⅔ dough, or leave covered in fridge and use when fresh croissants are required. Dough will keep for up to four days.

11. Glaze with milk and bake at 350°F for 30 minutes. Best eaten same day.

7

STARTERS, SOUPS AND SALADS

FRUIT COCKTAIL

Serves 4.

3g fiber/65 calories per glass.

1 grapefruit
1 lemon
1 orange
1 lime
1 small fresh pineapple, or can pineapple in own juice
Perrier or similar naturally sparkling mineral water

1. Cut pith and peel from the citrus fruits and roughly chop. Remove seeds. Place fruit in a blender.

2. Cut skin from the pineapple and remove central core if very woody. Chop and add to blender.

3. Liquidize fruits and place in a large jug. Cover.

4. Make the juice only just before serving to minimize vitamin loss. To cool, stir in ice cubes and add sparkling water to taste.

PERSIMMON COCKTAIL

Serves 4.
3½g fiber/80 calories per portion.

2 large persimmons
2 oranges
2 dessert pears
Orange juice

1. Remove stalks from the persimmons and roughly chop.

2. Peel the oranges and remove pith and seeds. Roughly chop.

3. Core the pears and chop.

4. Place all ingredients in a blender and blend to thick purée. Add a few ice cubes to mixture.

5. Add orange juice to achieve desired consistency for cocktail.

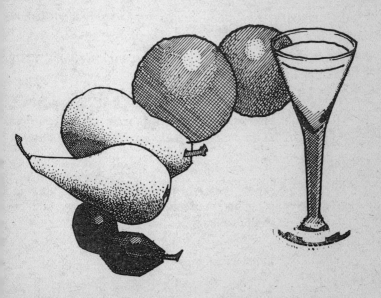

MELON SALAD
Serves 4.
5g fiber/100 calories per portion.

1 large canteloupe melon
1 papaya
2 cups sliced strawberries
2 oranges

1. Cut the melon in half. Remove seeds and reserve fruit.

2. Using a Parisienne cutter (melon baller) scoop balls from the flesh.

3. Halve the papaya and remove seeds. Slice thinly.

4. Arrange the melon balls, papaya and slices of strawberry on serving plates and pour over the freshly squeezed juice of 2 oranges.

5. Chill for 30 minutes before serving.

HUMMUS
Serves 4.
5½g fiber/390 calories per portion.

1 cup chickpeas
2 cloves garlic
Juice of 2 lemons
Sea salt
Freshly ground black pepper
Pinch cayenne pepper
⅔ cup tahini
Freshly chopped parsley

1. Soak the chickpeas overnight in water. Drain and place in a saucepan of boiling water and cook until tender — about one hour. Drain, cook and purée.

2. Peel and crush the garlic and add to the puréed chickpeas. Stir in lemon juice, seasoning and tahini to taste.

3. Place the hummus in a serving dish and garnish with parsley.

SUMMER OMELETTE
Serves 4.
8g fiber/290 calories per portion.

1 pound new potatoes
8 ounces young carrots
1⅓ cups peas
6 free-range eggs
Sea salt
Freshly ground black pepper
1 tablespoon freshly chopped basil
2½ tablespoons unsalted butter or corn oil

1. Scrub, but do not peel, the potatoes and carrots. Steam or boil until just cooked. Drain.

2. Cook the peas until just tender. Drain.

3. Dice the potatoes and carrots and mix with the peas.

4. Whisk eggs well and season. Stir in basil.

5. Place fat in a large omelette pan and allow butter to melt and foam, but not brown.

6. Pour in the omelette mixture. As it begins to set, lift edges with a spatula and allow unset mixture to run underneath and set.

7. Place the vegetables in the center of the omelette and cook for a minute or so. Fold the omelette in half to envelop the vegetables and carefully lift onto a serving plate. Cut into 4 and eat immediately. Alternatively make smaller omelettes.

GARDEN PEA SOUP
Serves 4.
11g fiber/140 calories per portion.

2 pounds fresh peas
1 bunch scallions
3¾ cups vegetable stock or water
1 tablespoon light cream
1 tablespoon chopped chives
Sea salt
Freshly ground black pepper

1. Shell the peas and place in a large saucepan.

2. Chop the scallions and add to the peas.

3. Add boiling stock or water. Simmer for about 20 minutes or until peas are cooked. Remove from heat.

4. When cool, sieve or purée in a blender.

5. Add cream, chives and seasoning to taste.

6. Good either hot or cold.

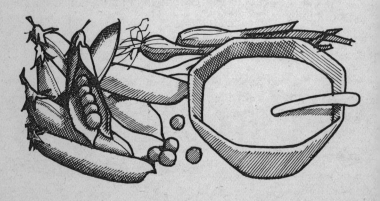

SUMMER VEGETABLE SOUP

Serves 4.
6½g fiber/220 calories per portion.

8 baby carrots
8 baby new potatoes, scrubbed
6 ounces tender young snap or green beans
1 bunch scallions
2 small zucchini, sliced
8 ounces fresh peas, shelled
2½ tablespoons unsalted butter or vegetable oil
3¾ cups vegetable stock or water
Sea salt
Freshly ground black pepper
Natural yogurt

1. Clean and roughly chop the first five vegetables and place with the peas in a saucepan with butter or oil. Cover and cook gently for 5 minutes.

2. Add stock or water and simmer for 15 minutes or until the vegetables are just cooked.

3. Season to taste and spoon equal amounts of each vegetable into each serving dish. Pour stock over.

4. Swirl a teaspoon of yogurt into each bowl of soup just before serving.

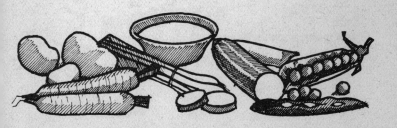

CELERIAC SOUP

Serves 4.
7g fiber/30 calories per portion.

1¼ cups chopped onion
⅔ cup chopped carrot
2⅔ cups chopped celeriac
2½ cups vegetable stock
Sea salt
Freshly ground black pepper

1. Place the onion and carrot in a heavy-based saucepan and sauté for five minutes.

2. Add the celeriac and stock. Cover and simmer for 20 minutes.

3. Purée the mixture in a blender and return to saucepan.

4. Season to taste and reheat.

5. Serve with home-made whole wheat bread for a satisfying meal and extra fiber.

WATERCRESS SOUP

Serves 4.
3½g fiber/90 calories per portion.

2 bunches watercress
12 ounces potatoes
1 onion
5 cups vegetable stock
Bouquet garni
Sea salt
Freshly ground black pepper

1. Wash the watercress well in plenty of cold water. Discard any yellowing leaves.

2. Scrub the potatoes and roughly chop.

3. Peel and dice the onion.

4. Place all the ingredients in a large saucepan with well-fitting lid and bring to the boil.

5. Lower heat and simmer for 15 minutes or until the vegetables are cooked.

6. Remove from heat and allow to cool slightly. Remove the bouquet garni and purée in a blender.

7. Chill before serving.

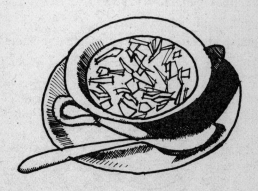

LENTIL SOUP

Serves 4.
6½g fiber/200 calories per portion.

1 cup lentils
1 teaspoon freshly grated ginger
½ teaspoon ground turmeric
1 teaspoon ground coriander
20 peppercorns and 20 cloves tied in muslin bag
5 cups water
2½ tablespoons unsalted butter
1 teaspoon cumin seeds
1 dried chili, diced
2 ripe tomatoes, diced

1. Pick over the lentils, removing all grit and stones and wash well.

2. Place the lentils, ginger, turmeric, coriander and muslin bag in a saucepan with water.

3. Bring to boil, lower heat and simmer for 30 minutes.

4. Melt the butter in a separate pan and add cumin seeds and chili. Sauté for 2 minutes being careful not to burn the butter.

5. Add the diced tomatoes and cook for further 2 minutes.

6. Remove bag from soup. Purée in a blender for smooth soup and return to pan.

7. Stir the tomato mixture into the soup and serve immediately.

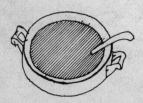

LEMON COLESLAW

Serves 4.
6g fiber/85 calories per portion.

½ small white cabbage, shredded
4 stalks celery, sliced
1 onion, diced
4 carrots, grated
1 eating apple, diced but not peeled
2½ tablespoons golden seedless raisins

Dressing:

2 tablespoons natural yogurt
Grated rind of ½ lemon
1 tablespoon freshly chopped parsley
Freshly ground black pepper

1. Place all the salad ingredients in a bowl and mix thoroughly.

2. Place the dressing ingredients in a screwtop jar and shake well.

3. Pour the dressing over the mixed salad and toss well.

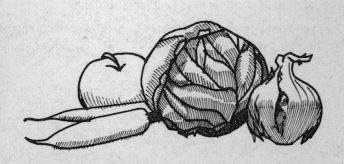

DATE AND WALNUT SALAD
Serves 4.
5½g fiber/ 240 calories per portion.

6 stalks celery, sliced
2 eating apples, diced but not peeled
Juice of ½ lemon
¾ cup English walnuts, chopped
⅔ cup chopped dates
1 cup cottage cheese

1. Toss the prepared celery and apple in lemon juice.

2. Add the nuts and dates to the apple mixture.

3. Stir in the cheese, and mix thoroughly.

KOHLRABI SALAD
Serves 4.
3g fiber/80 calories per portion.

1 pound kohlrabi
8 ounces carrots
2 medium onions
2 stalks celery
Salad dressing (page 51)

1. Scrub and grate the kohlrabi and carrot.

2. Peel and finely dice the onion and slice the celery.

3. Mix the salad dressing ingredients and pour over the prepared vegetables. Toss before serving.

GREEN BEAN AND CASHEW SALAD

Serves 4.
3½g fiber/220 calories per portion.

1 pound snap beans
1 cup cashew nuts
1 tablespoon cold-pressed safflower mayonnaise

1. Top and tail the beans and wash well.

2. Place the beans in a small amount of boiling water, cover and cook for 5 minutes. Drain and refresh with cold water.

3. Chop the cashews, or leave whole if preferred.

4. Toss the beans and cashews in mayonnaise and serve warm or cold.

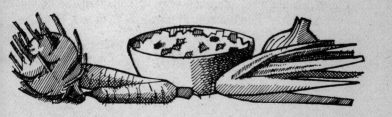

8.

LIGHT MEALS

MILLET BURGERS
Makes 4.
3½g fiber/240 calories per portion.

½ cup millet
1 cup diced onions
½ cup grated hard cheese
1 tablespoon chopped parsley
1 tablespoon stoneground mustard
2 free-range eggs, beaten
1 cup whole wheat breadcrumbs

1. Place the millet in a saucepan of boiling water. Cover and cook until soft, about 20 minutes. Drain.

2. Place the millet, onion, cheese, parsley, mustard ⅔ of the egg and half the breadcrumbs in a bowl and bind together into burger or large sausage shapes.

3. Roll the burgers in the beaten egg and coat in remaining breadcrumbs.

4. Lightly fry in a small amount of vegetable oil or bake in moderate oven on lightly oiled baking tray until golden brown. Turn once during cooking.

LENTIL BURGERS

Makes 4.
9g fiber/260 calories per burger.

1 cup lentils
2 stalks celery
1/2 cup grated white cabbage
1/2 cup ground almonds
1 1/2 cups fresh whole wheat breadcrumbs
2 tablespoons freshly chopped parsley
Pinch herb salt
Freshly ground black pepper
1 free-range egg

1. Pick over the lentils to remove grit and stones and place in a saucepan of boiling water. Cook for about 20 minutes or until soft. Drain if necessary.

2. Slice the celery.

3. Mix all ingredients (reserving 1/3 of the breadcrumbs) in a large bowl.

4. Form mixture into small burger shapes and roll in reserved breadcrumbs.

5. Smear a frying pan with oil and lightly fry for about 20 minutes, turning once. Alternatively, bake at 350°F, turning once, for 30 minutes.

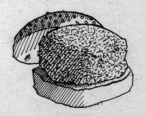

WALNUT BURGERS
Makes 4.
6g fiber/400 calories per burger.

1 cup ground walnuts
1 cup ground hazelnuts
2 cups fresh whole wheat breadcrumbs
1 onion, peeled and diced
Clove garlic, crushed
1 tablespoon freshly chopped parsley
1 teaspoon freshly chopped thyme or ⅓ dried
2 free-range eggs
Water to mix
⅓ cup sesame seeds

1. Place the nuts, breadcrumbs, onion, garlic and herbs in a mixing bowl and mix thoroughly.

2. Beat one egg with two tablespoons of water and stir into the nut mixture. Add more water, if necessary, to bind the mixture.

3. Shape into four burgers.

4. Beat the second egg and use to dip burgers in before rolling in sesame seeds.

5. Broil for 20 minutes, turning once. Alternatively bake on a lightly oiled baking tray for 20 minutes, turning once, at 375°F.

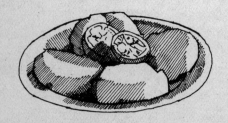

CURRIED PARSNIP BURGERS
Makes 4.
6g fiber/260 calories per burger.

1 pound parsnips
1 teaspoon garam masala or curry powder
1 teaspoon ground cumin
1 cup rolled oats
1 cup whole wheat breadcrumbs
1 free-range egg, beaten
1 tablespoon sesame seeds
1 tablespoon cumin seeds

1. Scrub and slice the parsnips. Steam or boil until cooked. Drain, reserving cooking liquid.

2. Mash the cooked parsnips using some of the cooking water to achieve a soft purée.

3. Mix garam masala and ground cumin into the mashed parsnips.

4. Stir in the oats and breadcrumbs.

5. Bind the mixture together with beaten egg and form into burger shapes.

6. Roll the burgers in mixed sesame and cumin seeds.

7. Lightly brush a heavy-based frying pan with oil and cook, turning once, for 20 minutes. Alternatively place on lightly oiled baking tray and bake at 350°F for 30 minutes until golden brown.

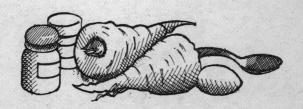

PARSNIP AND WALNUT FRITTERS
Makes 4.
9g fiber/340 calories per portion.

1½ pounds parsnips
⅔ cup skimmed milk
1 cup ground walnuts
½ cup whole wheat flour
2 free-range eggs
Sea salt
Freshly ground black pepper

1. Scrub and chop the parsnips. Steam or boil until cooked. Drain.

2. Add the milk to the parsnips, and purée.

3. Stir in the walnuts, flour, eggs and seasoning. Add more flour if necessary to make a stiff batter.

4. Smear a frying pan with oil and add tablespoons of mixture to form fritters. Turn once during cooking.

5. When cooked on both sides, remove and place on paper towels to remove any excess fat before serving.

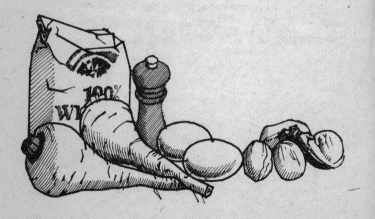

SAVORY SWEET POTATOES

Serves 4.
5g fiber/290 calories per portion.

2 large sweet potatoes
1 cup low-fat ricotta cheese
2 free-range egg yolks
4 shallots, finely diced
1 tablespoon chopped chives
Sea salt
Freshly ground black pepper

1. Scrub the potatoes and bake, unpeeled, at 400°F for 1 hour. Remove from oven.

2. Cut the potatoes in half and scoop out most of the flesh, leaving enough to hold the potato skin in shape.

3. Beat together the potato flesh, cheese, egg yolks, shallots and seasoning.

4. Pile mixture back into shells and return to oven to heat through.

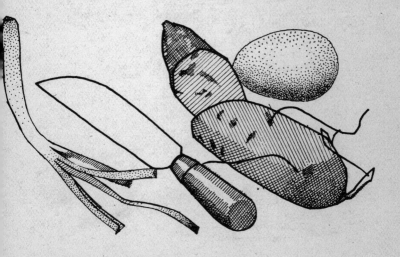

STILTON YAMS
Serves 4.
4½g fiber/260 calories per portion.

1½ pounds yam or sweet potato
⅔ cup skimmed milk
Freshly ground black pepper
1½ cup finely chopped watercress
1 cup Stilton or hard cheese of choice

1. Scrub the yams and slice into 1 in. thick rounds.

2. Place in a large, heavy-based saucepan with well-fitting lid and pour milk over them.

3. Season generously and place lid on pan. Simmer for 10 minutes until slices are just cooked. Drain.

4. Place the slices in a lightly oiled gratin dish and cover with watercress.

5. Pare thin slices of cheese, using a cheese plane and place on top of the watercress.

6. Grill until cheese is just melting.

7. Serve with home-made chutney.

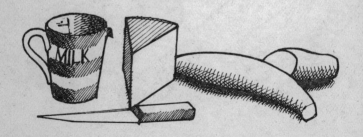

CHILI BAKED POTATOES

Serves 4.
19g fiber/360 calories per portion.

1⁄3 cups red kidney beans
4 large potatoes, scrubbed and baked in their skins
1 cup diced onion
2 fresh chilies, diced
1 teaspoon vegetable oil
1 8-ounce can tomatoes

1. Soak the beans overnight. Drain and boil in plenty of water for 45 minutes, or until soft.

2. While the beans are cooking bake the potatoes.

3. Sauté the onion in oil with the chilies.

4. Add the tomatoes and beans and simmer together for a further 15 minutes.

5. Remove the potatoes from oven. Cut a deep cross in tops, squeeze open and pour bean mixture over them.

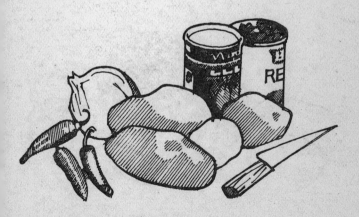

CABBAGE BAKED POTATOES

Serves 4.
8g fiber/240 calories per potato.

4 large potatoes, scrubbed and baked in their skins
2 cups shredded white cabbage
1⅓ cups grated cooking apples
⅔ cup golden seedless raisins
Sea salt
Freshly ground black pepper

1. While the potatoes are baking prepare the cabbage and apple and place in a large heavy-based saucepan with well-fitting lid.

2. Add a little water and cover. Cook gently for 30 minutes.

3. After 10 minutes add the raisins. Season to taste.

4. Remove the cooked potatoes from oven. Halve, and spoon cabbage mixture over.

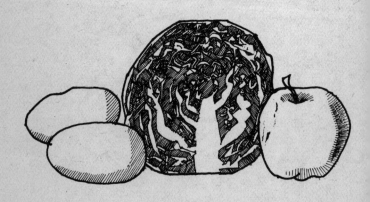

BROAD BEAN MINESTRONE

Serves 4.
6g fiber/140 calories per portion.

2 pounds broad beans
2 tablespoons olive oil
²/₃ cup diced onion
²/₃ cup diced carrot
1 stalk celery, chopped
5 cups vegetable stock
Pinch sea salt
2 cups whole wheat spaghetti broken into small pieces
Parmesan cheese (optional)

1. Shell the beans.

2. Heat oil in a saucepan and add the onion, carrot and celery. Cover and sauté for 5 minutes.

3. Add the beans and stock and bring to boil. Lower heat to simmering point for 20 minutes.

4. Stir in the spaghetti and simmer for further 10 minutes or until spaghetti is *al dente* (cooked, but still firm when bitten).

5. Serve at once, with a bowl of cheese for those who want it.

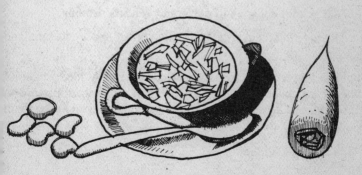

BRUSSELS SPROUTS LASAGNE

Serves 4.
5½g fiber/386 calories per portion.

8 ounces whole wheat lasagne
1 tablespoon corn oil
1⅓ cups diced onion
1 pound brussels sprouts
1¼ cups vegetable stock
½ teaspoon ground nutmeg
Sea salt
Freshly ground black pepper
2 cups natural yogurt
¾ cup chopped English walnuts
1 cup cottage cheese
2 free-range eggs, beaten

1. Boil the lasagne in plenty of water for 12 minutes or until *al dente* (still firm to the teeth when bitten, but just cooked). Drain, rinse in cold water and separate sheets.

2. Place oil in saucepan and add the onions. Cover and sauté for 5 minutes.

3. Clean and chop the brussels sprouts. Add to the onion with stock and seasoning. Cover and cook for 15 minutes or until sprouts are tender.

4. Purée sprout mixture in a blender or rub through a sieve.

5. Add ⅓ of the yogurt to purée and adjust seasoning.

6. Mix together the rest of the yogurt, cottage cheese, walnuts and eggs.

7. Place a layer of sprout mixture in base of a lightly oiled ovenproof dish and cover with lasagne. Place a layer of yogurt mixture on top. Repeat layers until sauces and pasta are used up, ending with yogurt mixture.

3. Bake at 400°F for 35-40 minutes, until topping is golden brown and set.

BROAD BEAN TAGLIATELLI

Serves 4.
10g fiber/270 calories per portion.

⅓ cup olive oil
2 cloves garlic, crushed
  dried chilli, chopped
  tablespoon freshly chopped parsley
1⅓ cups vegetable stock
2 cups shelled broad beans
⅓ cups shelled fresh peas
½ cups whole wheat tagliatelli

1. Place the olive oil, garlic, chilli and parsley in a saucepan. Cover and sauté for 5 minutes.

2. Add the stock, beans and peas. Cover and simmer for 20 minutes.

3. Boil the tagliatelli in plenty of salted (optional) water for 12 minutes, or until *al dente* (that is, still firm to the teeth when bitten, but just cooked). Drain.

4. Place the tagliatelli on serving dish and pour bean sauce over it.

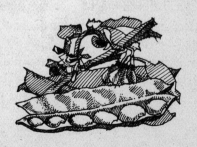

LASAGNE

Serves 4.
12g fiber/300 calories per portion.

8 ounces whole wheat lasagne
¼ cup whole wheat flour
2½ tablespoons unsalted butter or polyunsaturated margarine
⅔ cup vegetable stock
1 cup cooked chopped spinach
Freshly ground nutmeg, to taste
Freshly ground black pepper
1⅓ cups diced onion
1 clove garlic, crushed
1 pound tomatoes, chopped
1 medium red pepper, diced
⅔ cup diced carrots
¾ cup chopped cashew nuts
1 tablespoon basil
1 tablespoon oregano
Freshly ground black pepper

1. Place the lasagne in saucepan with plenty of boiling water and cook for about 12 minutes, or until *al dente* (cooked, but still firm to the teeth when bitten). Drain and separate sheets.

2. Place the flour and butter in saucepan and cook together, stirring continuously over a low heat.

3. Gradually add the vegetable stock, stirring all the time as the sauce thickens.

4. Stir in the spinach and seasoning.

5. In another saucepan place the onion and garlic. Cover and sauté for 5 minutes.

6. Add the tomatoes, pepper and carrots. Cover and cook for a further 10 minutes. Stir in the nuts, herbs and seasoning to taste.

7. Lightly oil an ovenproof dish and place a layer of the tomato mixture in the base. Cover with a layer of lasagne.

8. On top of the lasagne place a layer of the spinach mixture and top with more lasagne. Repeat once more, ending with spinach mixture.

9. Bake at 375°F for 30 minutes. Serve with a green salad.

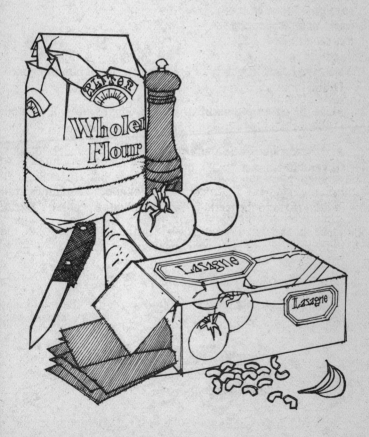

SPAGHETTI WITH LIMA BEANS

Serves 4.
18g fiber/270 calories per portion.

1⅓ cups lima beans
1⅓ cups diced onion
2 cloves garlic, crushed
1 tablespoon olive oil
1 pound tomatoes, roughly chopped
2 stalks celery, finely sliced
⅔ cup vegetable stock
Bouquet garni
2 tablespoons freshly chopped parsley
8 ounces whole wheat spaghetti
1 large carrot, grated

1. Boil the beans in plenty of boiling water until almost cooked. Drain.

2. Place the onion and garlic in a heavy-based saucepan with oil. Cover with a well-fitting lid and sauté for 5 minutes.

3. Add the tomatoes, beans, celery, stock, bouquet garni and parsley. Cover and simmer for 20 minutes.

4. Boil the spaghetti in plenty of water for about 12 minutes until *al dente* (firm to the teeth when bitten, but just cooked). Drain.

5. Place spaghetti in a serving dish. Stir the grated carrot into the bean mixture and pour over spaghetti.

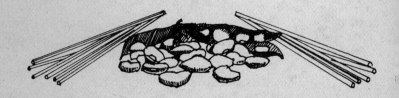

FENNEL PASTA

Serves 4.
12g fiber/350 calories per portion.

2 large fennel bulbs, diced
1⅓ cups diced onion
1 large red pepper, diced
1 tablespoon olive oil
⅔ cup vegetable stock
⅔ cup raisins
1 cup slivered almonds
Sea salt
Freshly ground black pepper
4 cups whole wheat pasta shells

1. Place the fennel, onion and pepper in a saucepan with the oil. Cover with a well-fitting lid and sauté over low heat for 10 minutes.

2. Add stock, raisins, almonds and seasoning. Cover and simmer for 20 minutes.

3. While this is cooking boil the pasta in a large saucepan with plenty of boiling water for about 12 minutes, or until *al dente* (that is, still firm when bitten, but just cooked). Drain.

4. Place the pasta in a serving dish and cover with fennel sauce. Toss well and serve.

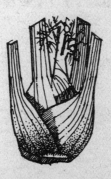

BEAN AND PASTA SALAD

Serves 4.
10g fiber/260 calories per portion.

½ cup red kidney beans
½ cup black-eye peas
3 cups whole wheat pasta shells
1 small can soyaprotein frankfurters

Dressing:

2 tablespoons olive oil
1 tablespoon wine vinegar
1 teaspoon stoneground mustard
Freshly ground black pepper

1. Place the beans and black-eyed peas in a saucepan of boiling water
    and boil fiercely for at least 10 minutes. Continue cooking until
    soft — about 45 minutes. Drain and cool.

2. Place the pasta shells in boiling water and cook for about 12
    minutes until *al dente* (still slightly firm when bitten, but just
    cooked). Drain and cool.

3. If the frankfurters are not ready to eat, cook according to
    manufacturer's instructions and allow to cool.

4. Combine the dressing ingredients in a screwtop jar and shake well.

5. Place all salad ingredients in serving bowl and toss in dressing.

9

MAIN MEALS

ADUKI ROAST
Serves 4.
6g fiber/390 calories per portion.

2 cups cooked aduki beans
²/₃ cup tomato sauce (page 104)
1 cup ground English walnuts
1 cup ground peanuts
¾ cup rolled oats
2 cups whole wheat breadcrumbs
1¹/₃ cups finely diced onion
²/₃ cup finely grated carrot
1 tablespoon freshly chopped parsley
2 free-range eggs

1. Place the cooked beans in a blender with a few tablespoons of tomato sauce, and purée.

2. Add the rest of the ingredients and blend together. For a rougher texture mix puréed beans in a bowl with the other ingredients. Use chopped nuts rather than ground nuts, if preferred.

3. Turn the mixture into a lightly oiled loaf tin and bake at 375°F for 1 hour.

CURRIED SPLIT PEAS
Serves 4.
10g fiber/300 calories per portion.

1 cup split peas
1 tablespoon vegetable oil
1⅓ cup diced onion
1 teaspoon ground cumin
1 teaspoon ground coriander
2 dried chillies, chopped
1 clove garlic, crushed
2 apples, cored and diced, but not peeled
1 teaspoon lemon juice
8 ounces tomatoes, chopped
⅔ cup golden seedless raisins
2 cups vegetable stock

1. Cook the split peas in plenty of boiling water for 30 minutes.

2. Sauté the onion, cumin, coriander, chillies and garlic in oil in heavy-based saucepan with well-fitting lid, for 5 minutes.

3. Add the apples, lemon juice, tomatoes, raisins, split peas and stock and bring to simmering point.

4. Replace the lid and simmer for 10 minutes.

5. Serve hot with brown rice.

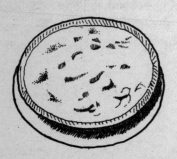
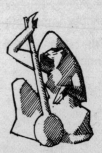

EILEEN'S GROUNDNUT STEW AND MANGOS

Serves 4.
13g fiber/470 calories per portion.

1⅓ cups diced onion
1 fresh chilli, finely chopped
½ teaspoon grated fresh ginger
1 teaspoon vegetable oil
1 pound tomatoes (canned or fresh)
2 cups crunchy peanut butter
1 pound eggplants
4 ounces okra
2 mangos
2 bananas

1. Place the onion, chilli and ginger in a heavy-based saucepan. Add oil, cover with a well-fitting lid and sauté gently for 5 minutes.

2. Stir in the tomatoes and break them up with back of spoon.

3. Add the peanut butter and simmer for 20 minutes.

4. Meanwhile wash and dice the unpeeled eggplants and steam or boil for 20 minutes.

5. Wash and remove stems from the okra. Steam or boil for 10 minutes.

6. Stir the eggplants and okra into the peanut mixture and continue cooking for 5 minutes.

7. Peel and slice the mangos and bananas and mix together.

8. Serve the groundnut stew and offer the bananas and mangos separately. Best served with brown rice.

PECAN ROAST

Serves 4.
8g fiber/600 calories per portion.

2 cups pecan nuts
4 cups whole wheat breadcrumbs
1⅓ cups finely diced onion
1⅓ cups finely grated carrot
1 tablespoon freshly chopped sage or ⅓ dried
Juice of ½ lemon
Sea salt
Freshly ground black pepper
2 free-range eggs

1. Grind or chop the pecan nuts, depending on preferred texture of the roast.

2. Stir in the breadcrumbs, onion, carrot, sage, lemon juice and seasoning.

3. Add the beaten eggs to bind the mixture. If more liquid is needed use a little vegetable stock.

4. Turn the mixture into a lightly oiled loaf tin and bake at 375°F for 45 minutes.

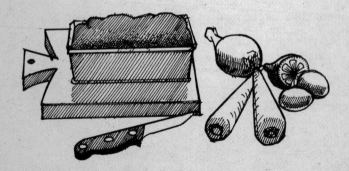

WHOLE WHEAT PANCAKES
Makes 10.
2½g fiber/75 calories per pancake.

1 cup whole wheat flour
Pinch sea salt (optional)
1 free-range egg, beaten
1⅓ cups skimmed milk or ⅔ cup milk and ⅔ cup water

1. Sieve the flour and salt into a mixing bowl.

2. Make a well in center and add the egg.

3. Stir flour into the liquid working from the center towards the sides of bowl. Keep the paste smooth and avoid lumps by working slowly.

4. Gradually add milk to mixture, and beat well when all liquid is worked in.

5. To ensure light pancakes use a heavy-based omelette pan. Heat a smear of oil in the pan before adding mixture and pour only enough batter in to cover the base of the pan when the mixture is thinly spread.

6. Turn the pancakes once after loosening with flexible spatula.

Note: To make a complete meal out of pancakes, see the following recipes for exciting fillings.

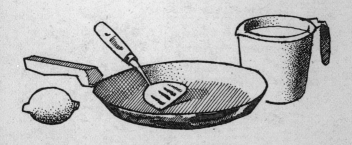

SPINACH PANCAKES

Makes 10.
6g fiber/145 calories per pancake.

1 box frozen spinach, or 1 pound fresh spinach
1 tablespoon whole wheat flour
1 tablespoon unsalted butter or polyunsaturated margarine
²/₃ cup skim milk
Grated fresh nutmeg
Pinch sea salt
Freshly ground black pepper
¾ cup grated hard cheese of choice

1. Make the pancakes (page 75).

2. Wash fresh spinach in plenty of cold water to remove all dirt and grit. Slice with a sharp knife.

3. Place in a large saucepan and cover with a well-fitting lid. Cook for about 5 minutes, turning once or twice. There is no need to add more water to cook the spinach in. If using frozen spinach, drain well after defrosting, then heat gently.

4. Add the flour and butter or margarine to the spinach and stir in well.

5. Gradually add milk, stirring continuously, to thicken mixture.

6. Season to taste and divide the mixture into equal amounts for each pancake. Roll up the pancakes and place in an ovenproof dish.

7. Sprinkle cheese over the pancakes and bake at 350°F for 20 minutes.

BROCCOLI AND CASHEW PANCAKES

Makes 10.
4g fiber/100 calories per pancake.

8 ounces broccoli spears
1/2 cup cashew nuts, finely chopped
1 tablespoon freshly chopped parsley
1/3 cup ground coconut
2/3 cup natural yogurt
1 free-range egg, beaten
Sea salt
Freshly ground black pepper

1. Make the pancakes (page 75).

2. Steam or boil the broccoli for 4 minutes in minimum amount of water.

3. Mix the nuts, parsley, coconut, natural yogurt and egg together in a bowl.

4. Place some broccoli on each pancake and spoon the nut mixture over. Roll the pancakes up.

5. Place the pancakes in a lightly oiled ovenproof dish. Cover and bake at 375°F for 25-30 minutes.

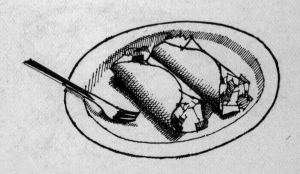

AVOCADO AND BRAZIL PANCAKES
Makes 10.
4g fiber/270 calories per pancake.

2 ripe avocados
1/2 lemon
1/2 cup finely chopped Brazil nuts
2 tablespoons freshly chopped parsley
3/4 cup chopped tomatoes
1/2 cup whole wheat breadcrumbs
2 tablespoons tomato sauce (page 104)

1. Peel and slice the avocados. Dress with lemon juice to prevent browning.

2. Mix together the nuts, parsley, tomatoes and breadcrumbs and stir in the avocado slices.

3. Add tomato sauce to bind and place a tablespoon of mixture on each pancake. Roll up.

4. Place the pancakes in an ovenproof dish and cover. Bake at 400°F for 15 minutes.

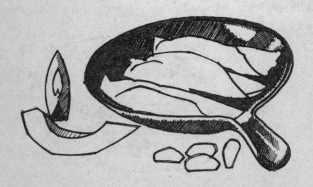

TOPPED VEGETABLES

Serves 4.
9g fiber/280 calories per portion.

1⅓ cups diced rutabaga
1⅓ cups sliced carrots
1⅓ cups shelled peas
2 tablespoons chopped parsley
1⅓ cups vegetable stock

Topping:

2½ tablespoons unsalted butter or polyunsaturated margarine
¼ cup mashed potato
½ cup grated hard cheese of choice
½ cup oatmeal
1 cup whole wheat flour
Sea salt
Freshly ground black pepper
1 tablespoon skim milk

1. Steam or boil the rutabaga and carrots for 5 minutes. Blanch the peas for 1 minute.

2. Mix the vegetables with the parsley and stock and place in an ovenproof dish.

3. Cream the fat and potato together.

4. Mix the cheese, oatmeal, flour and seasoning and add to the potato.

5. Add enough water to form a soft dough and roll out. Carefully lift it onto the vegetables to form a pastry-style crust.

6. Glaze with milk and bake at 400°F for 30 minutes.

MOUSSAKA
Serves 4.
10g fiber/670 calories per portion.

1 pound eggplants
1 tablespoon olive oil
2 cups diced onion
1 clove garlic, crushed
1 pound tomatoes, chopped
2 tablespoons freshly chopped parsley
2 cups crunchy peanut butter
²/₃ cup tomato sauce (page 104)
Sea salt
Freshly ground black pepper

Topping:

2¹/₂ tablespoon polyunsaturated margarine
¹/₄ cup whole wheat flour
1¹/₃ cups skimmed milk
¹/₂ cup rolled oats
Pinch sea salt (optional)
Freshly ground black pepper
³/₄ cup grated hard cheese of choice
2 free-range eggs, separated

1. Wash and slice the eggplants. Blanch in boiling water for 3 minutes. Drain.

2. Heat half the oil in large non-stick frying pan and sauté the eggplants for 10 minutes, turning once.

3. In another pan sauté the onions and garlic for 5 minutes.

4. Add the tomatoes to the onions, plus the parsley and stir in the peanut butter and tomato sauce. Heat through.

5. Place a layer of eggplants in an ovenproof dish. Top with a layer of tomato mixture and repeat until the mixture is used up. Set aside.

6. To make a topping, place the fat and flour in a heavy-based saucepan over low heat and make a *roux* by stirring continuously.

7. Gradually add milk, still stirring to prevent lumps forming.

8. When all the liquid has been added remove from heat and stir in the oats and seasoning.

9. Add the cheese and egg yolks.

10. Whisk egg whites to firm peaks and quickly fold into the mixture.

11. Pour immediately over vegetable mixture and bake at 375°F for 40 minutes or until topping is risen and golden.

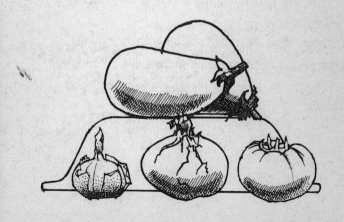

TOMATO AND OLIVE PIZZA

Serves 4.
8½g fiber/250 calories per portion.

Dough:

2 cups whole wheat flour
2 teaspoons fresh yeast
⅔ cup warm water
1 teaspoon vegetable oil
½ vitamin C tablet, crushed

Topping:

1 16-ounce can tomatoes
1⅓ cups diced onion
1 clove garlic, crushed
1 large red pepper, seeded and diced
⅔ cup grated carrot
2 tablespoons freshly chopped parsley
½ cup pitted black olives
Freshly ground black pepper
½ cup mozzarella cheese

1. Sieve the flour and salt into a bowl.

2. Crumble the yeast into warm water and stir in the oil and vitamin C tablet.

3. Pour the water onto the flour and mix to a dough.

4. Turn onto a floured surface and knead for 5 minutes.

5. Return the dough to the bowl and cover. Leave to rest for 10 minutes.

6. Place the tomatoes in a saucepan over low heat and break up with a fork. Add the onion, garlic, pepper and carrot and cook for 10 minutes, or until nicely thickened.

7. Stir in the parsley, remove from heat and season to taste.

8. Return the pizza dough to the floured surface and roll out. Place on a large pizza pan, or make 4 smaller rounds and place on a lightly oiled baking tray.

9. Spread the tomato mixture on top of dough and arrange the olives on the mixture.

10. Slice the mozzarella thinly and place on top of the pizza. Bake at 400°F for 25 minutes.

Alternative toppings: A small can of anchovy fillets can be added to the tomato sauce. Sliced mushrooms can be added to the mixture, or as decoration. Tuna fish goes well with pizza toppings.

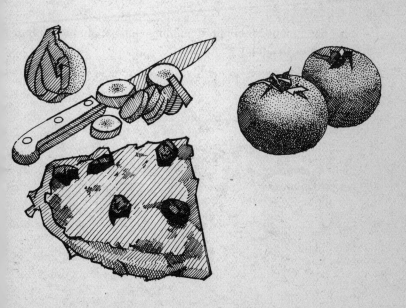

PEASE PUDDING

Serves 4.
6g fiber/210 calories per portion.

1 cup yellow split peas
²/₃ cup diced onion
1 bay leaf
2½ cups vegetable stock
1 teaspoon freshly chopped sage or ⅓ dried
2½ tablespoons polyunsaturated margarine
1 free-range egg

1. Pour hot water over the peas and soak overnight. Drain.

2. Place the peas in a saucepan with the onion, bay leaf, stock and sage. Cover. Bring to boil and simmer for 1½ hours until peas are cooked. Watch the pot to ensure it does not boil dry and burn. Add water if necessary.

3. When the peas are cooked, cool and purée in a blender with the seasoning, margarine and egg.

4. Turn the mixture into a lightly oiled pudding mold and cover with parchment paper and a pudding cloth or aluminum foil. Secure and steam for 45 minutes.

5. Turn out and serve hot with vegetables or cold with salad.

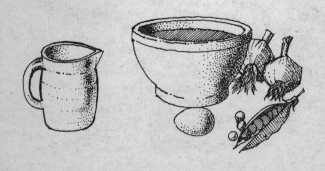

BAKED NUT CABBAGE

Serves 4.
7g fiber/280 calories per portion.

1½ pounds green cabbage
Freshly ground black pepper
¼ cup unsalted butter or polyunsaturated margarine
⅔ cup vegetable stock
Pinch ground mace
⅓ cup salted peanuts
½ cup grated hard cheese of choice

1. Using a sharp knife shred the cabbage finely and wash well.

2. Heat a little water in large saucepan. When boiling, drop in the cabbage and season with pepper. Simmer for 5 minutes. Drain, reserving liquid.

3. In another saucepan melt the butter and flour, stirring well to make a *roux*. Gradually stir in the vegetable stock and enough water from the cabbage to make a creamy sauce. Season with mace.

4. Lightly oil an ovenproof dish and place a layer of cabbage in the bottom.

5. Cover with a little sauce and sprinkle some nuts and cheese on top of the sauce. Repeat the process, ending with a cheese layer.

6. Bake at 400°F for 15 minutes.

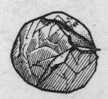

STIR-FRY VEGETABLES
Serves 4.
5½g fiber/270 calories per portion.

1 cup brown rice
2 leeks
1 large onion
1 tablespoon sesame oil
1 green pepper
10 ounces canned bamboo shoots
2 cups beansprouts

1. Wash the rice and place in a saucepan with 2½ times its volume of boiling water. Cover and simmer for 40 minutes.

2. Scrub and slice the leeks.

3. Peel and dice the onion and place, with the leek, in a wok, or frying pan with the oil. Sauté for 3 minutes.

4. Wash and seed the pepper. Dice and add to wok.

5. Drain the bamboo shoots. Slice thinly and add to wok.

6. Wash the beansprouts and, just before serving, stir into vegetables. Allow to heat through and serve hot with the rice and Sweet and Sour Sauce if liked (page 88).

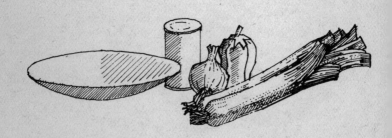

STIR-FRY VEGETABLES AND BEANS

Serves 4.
5g fiber/360 calories per portion.

1 cup brown rice
1 tablespoon sesame oil
1 large onion, diced
1 clove garlic, crushed
2 carrots, cut into matchsticks
1 large head broccoli, divided into florets
1 red pepper, seeded and cut into strips
1 cup cooked black-eyed peas

1. Wash the rice and put it in a saucepan with 2½ times its volume of water. Cover and bring to boil. Cook for 40 minutes.

2. Heat the oil in a wok and sauté the onion and garlic for 5 minutes.

3. Add the other vegetables, stirring all the time to prevent sticking and help even cooking.

4. Just before serving stir in the black-eyed peas and heat through.

5. Serve with Sweet and Sour Sauce (page 88).

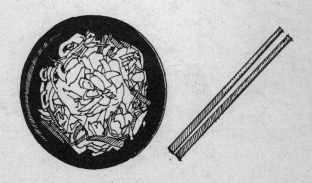

SWEET AND SOUR SAUCE
0g fiber/196 calories total.

1 orange
2 tablespoons red wine vinegar
1 tablespoon raw sugar
2 tablespoons tomato paste
2 tablespoons water
2 tablespoons soy sauce

1. Cut the orange in half and squeeze juice.

2. Place juice with all the other ingredients in saucepan and heat gently until all ingredients are thoroughly combined.

3. Pour over Stir-fry vegetables (pages 86 and 87).

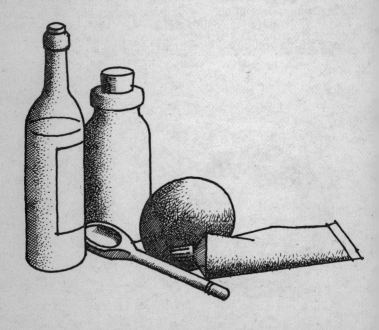

WHOLE WHEAT PASTRY FLAN CASE
3½g fiber/260 calories.

1½ cups whole wheat flour
⅓ cup polyunsaturated margarine
1 free-range egg yolk, beaten
Water to mix

1. Sieve the flour into a mixing bowl.

2. Rub in fat until the mixture resembles breadcrumbs in texture.

3. Make a well in the center and stir in the yolk and water to make a soft dough.

4. Turn onto a floured surface and roll out.

5. Carefully fold in half and lift into a lightly oiled flan ring or ceramic flan dish.

6. Place a layer of parchment paper on top of the pastry and fill with baking beans. Bake blind at 400°F for 10 minutes.

7. Remove from oven and lift out the paper and beans. The pastry case is now ready for filling.

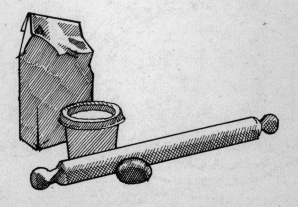

ONION TART

Serves 4.
4½g fiber/359 calories per portion.

1⅔ cups diced onion
½ cup ricotta cheese
⅔ cup natural yogurt
2 free-range eggs
Sea salt (optional)
Freshly ground black pepper
Pinch of ground mace
Baked blind pastry case (page 89)

1. Place the onions in a frying pan smeared with a little vegetable oil, and sauté for 5 minutes.

2. Beat together the cheese, yogurt, eggs and seasoning.

3. Put the onions onto absorbent paper to drain off any excess fat, and turn them into the prepared pastry case.

4. Pour the yogurt mixture on top and bake at 400°F for 35 minutes or until golden brown and set.

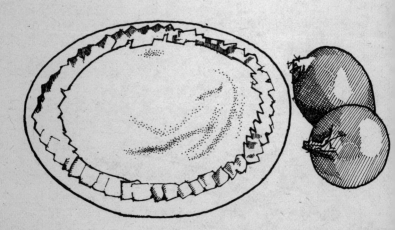

LEEK AND POTATO QUICHE
Serves 4.
7g fiber/390 calories per portion.

12 ounces potatoes
8 ounces leeks
²/₃ cup natural yogurt
1 free-range egg, separated
Sea salt
Freshly ground black pepper
Baked blind pastry case (page 89)

1. Scrub the potatoes and dice, but do not peel. You should have about 3¼ cups.

2. Slice the leeks and wash well.

3. Place the potatoes and leeks in a saucepan with a smear of vegetable oil. Cover and cook for 5 minutes.

4. Beat together the yogurt, egg yolk and seasoning.

5. Place the leeks and potatoes on absorbent paper to remove any excess oil, then turn into the prepared pastry case.

6. Whisk the egg white to stiff peaks and fold into the yogurt mixture.

7. Pour over the top of the vegetables in the pastry case and bake at 375°F for 35 minutes or until golden brown and firm to the touch.

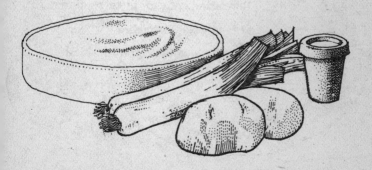

CHILLI BEANS
Serves 4.
20g fiber/260 calories per portion.

1²/₃ cups kidney beans, soaked overnight
1 tablespoon vegetable oil
8 ounces green pepper, seeded and diced
²/₃ cup diced onion
2 cloves garlic, crushed
4 fresh chillis, seeded and finely diced
1 pound canned tomatoes
²/₃ cup vegetable stock
1½ teaspoon ground cumin
1 teaspoon oregano
Sea salt (optional)
8 ounces broccoli, divided into florets

1. Drain the soaked beans and put them in a saucepan of boiling water. Cook for about 40 minutes, or until soft.

2. Heat the oil in a heavy-based saucepan.

3. Add the pepper, onion, garlic and chillies and sauté, covered, for 10 minutes.

4. Add the tomatoes and break them up with a wooden spoon.

5. Add the vegetable stock and cook for a further 10 minutes.

6. Stir in cumin, oregano and salt.

7. Add the broccoli florets and cook for further 5 minutes.

8. Stir in the cooked beans. Heat through.

9. Serve with brown rice for a complete protein meal.

SWEET AND SOUR KOHLRABI

Serves 4.
4g fiber/70 calories each.

4 kohlrabi, evenly sized
1 large green pepper
1 large yellow or red pepper
1 leek
1 tablespoon sesame oil
Sweet and Sour Sauce (page 88)

1. Scrub the kohlrabi and place the whole vegetables in a large saucepan of boiling water. Cook for about 30 minutes.

2. Scrub and dice the peppers. Clean and slice the leek.

3. Heat the oil in a large, heavy-based saucepan or frying pan and add the peppers and leek. Stir them while cooking for about 5 minutes, until they are just cooked.

4. Pour the sweet and sour sauce over the vegetables and cover. Place in oven to keep warm.

5. Drain the kohlrabi and slice off the tops. Scoop out the center and fill with sweet and sour vegetables. Replace the tops and serve.

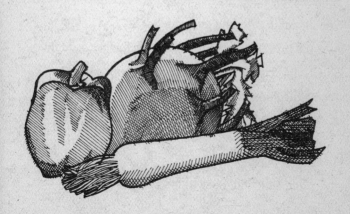

BROWN RICE RING

Serves 4.
4½g fiber/400 calories per portion.

1½ cups brown rice
1 red pepper
1 yellow or green pepper
¼ cup sunflower seeds
½ cup pine nuts

1. Place the washed rice in 3¾ cups of boiling water, cover and cook until soft — about 40 minutes.

2. Scrub and finely dice the peppers.

3. Put the rice in a mixing bowl when cooked and stir in the diced peppers. Add the sunflower seeds and pine nuts.

4. Rinse a savarin mold with cold water and pour water away.

5. Press the rice mixture into the wet mold. By pressing the mixture down firmly the rice will take shape when the mold is removed.

6. Chill in the fridge before use.

7. To unmold, place a serving dish on top of mold and invert, supporting plate. If the rice does not come away easily slip a sharp knife around sides, invert and tap the top gently when inverted.

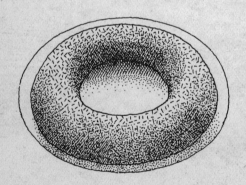

ʼARSNIP CHEESE

erves 4.

g fiber/350 calories per portion.

pounds parsnips
cup unsalted butter or polyunsaturated margarine
cups whole wheat breadcrumbs
cup grated hard cheese of choice

Scrub the parsnips and chop roughly.

Put them in a large saucepan and boil or steam until just cooked.

Drain and mash with a potato masher, mixing in margarine or butter.

Stir in the breadcrumbs and cheese and place in a lightly oiled ovenproof dish.

Make a pattern on top with a fork and broil for a few minutes, or bake in a moderate oven, until top is golden brown and mixture has heated through.

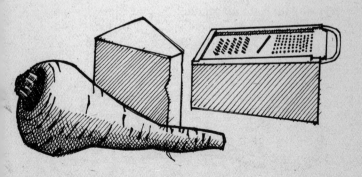

PARSNIP AND TOMATO BAKE

Serves 4.
7g fiber/500 calories per portion.

2 pounds parsnips
1 pound tomatoes
¼ cup unsalted butter or polyunsaturated margarine
Sea salt
Freshly ground black pepper
1½ cups Edam or 1 cup grated Gruyère
⅔ cup light cream
1 cup whole wheat breadcrumbs

1. Scrub the parsnips and cut into strips.

2. Place in a lightly oiled pan with well fitting lid and sweat for 5 minutes.

3. Place the tomatoes in boiling water for 1 minute. Drain and transfer to cold water. Slit the skins which should now be easily removed. Slice tomatoes thinly.

4. Lightly oil an ovenproof dish with some of the fat.

5. Put a layer of parsnips in the base, cover with a layer of tomatoes. Season and sprinkle with a little cheese and cream.

6. Repeat layers, reserving a little cheese. Mix the cheese with breadcrumbs and use as topping.

7. Bake at 350°F for 40 minutes.

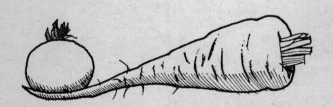

CHICKPEA AND SQUASH HOTPOT

Serves 4.
9½g fiber/500 calories per portion.

1 cup hummus (page 44, halve the quantities)
1 large summer squash
1 pound new potatoes
1 bunch scallions
4 baby carrots

1. Wash the squash and slice into thick rounds, removing the seeds.

2. Lightly oil a large casserole and arrange the rings inside.

3. Fill the rings with hummus.

4. Scrub the potatoes and place, whole, around the rings.

5. Wash and trim the scallions. Cut into short lengths and add to the casserole.

6. Scrub the carrots and place in the casserole with two or three tablespoons water.

7. Cover and bake at 375°F for 30 minutes.

Note: It should not be necessary to add more water or vegetable stock because the squash will produce its own and will cook in its own steam. However, check during cooking to make sure the dish is not burning and add water or stock if necessary.

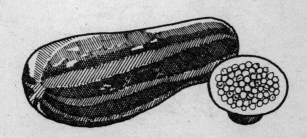

TOMATO BEANS
Serves 4.
14g fiber/150 calories per portion.

1 cup navy beans
1 pound canned tomatoes
2 stalks celery, diced
Rind of 1 orange
Bouquet garni

1. Pour boiling water over the beans and soak overnight. Rinse and place in a saucepan with boiling water and cook for about 1 hour or until soft. Using a pressure cooker will cut the time down to about 30 minutes.

2. While the beans are cooking place the tomatoes in a saucepan with the celery and pared orange rind and bouquet garni. Break up the tomatoes with a wooden spoon.

3. Cook the tomato mixture over low heat for 25 minutes. Remove the bouquet garni and orange rind and press through sieve or purée in a blender.

4. Drain the beans and stir into the tomato sauce.

5. Thicken if preferred with potato flour or arrowroot dissolved in water.

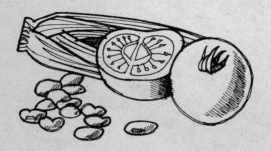

TOMATO BEAN BALLS

Serves 4.
6g fiber/250 calories per portion.

1 cup cooked black-eyed peas
1 cup ground hazelnuts
1 tablespoon tahini
1 thick slice whole wheat bread
8 ounces canned tomatoes
Sea salt
Freshly ground black pepper
1 orange
1 tablespoon tomato paste

1. Place the beans in a food processor with the nuts and tahini.

2. Make breadcrumbs from the slice of bread and add to beans.

3. Drain tomatoes and add the pulp only to the food processor, reserve the juice. Blend all the ingredients in the food processor.

4. Remove from processor and season to taste. Add grated rind of well-washed orange.

5. Form the bean mixture into balls and place on a lightly oiled baking tray. Bake at 400°F for 30 minutes.

6. To make the sauce place juice from tomatoes, juice from orange and tomato purée in saucepan. Heat through and dilute, if preferred, with water.

7. Pour the sauce over the hot bean balls and serve at once.

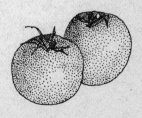

PASTA NIÇOISE
Serves 2.
4½g fiber/145 calories per portion.

½ red pepper
1 clove garlic
3 shallots
4 tomatoes
2 cups whole wheat pasta shells
1¼ cups water or vegetable stock
¼ cup black olives
1 tablespoon freshly chopped parsley
1 tablespoon freshly chopped chives
1 tablespoon tomato ketchup
1 small can anchovy fillets

1. Wash and dice the red pepper. Place in a lightly oiled saucepan.

2. Crush the garlic, dice shallots and chop the tomatoes and add to saucepan. Cover and cook over low heat for 5 minutes.

3. While the vegetables are cooking, place the pasta in a saucepan of boiling water and cook for about 12 minutes or until *al dente* (still firm to the teeth when bitten, but just cooked).

4. Add stock to the tomato mixture and stir in the olives, herbs, ketchup and anchovies. Continue to cook for 5 minutes.

5. Drain the pasta and place in a serving dish. Pour on the tomato sauce and serve at once.

DOLMAS

Serves 4.
9g fiber/350 calories per portion.

8 large outer leaves of cabbage
1 tablespoon olive oil
1⅓ cups diced onion
1 clove garlic, crushed
1 pound celeriac, diced
3½ tablespoons sunflower seeds
½ cupful pine nuts
⅓ cup golden seedless raisins
1⅓ cups cooked brown rice
1¼ cups tomato sauce (page 104)

1. Clean the cabbage leaves and blanch in boiling water. Drain, reserving liquid.

2. Place the oil in a saucepan and add the onion and garlic. Sauté for 5 minutes.

3. Add the celeriac and sunflower seeds. Cover and cook for 5 minutes over low heat.

4. Stir in pine nuts, sultanas and rice. Heat through.

5. Spread the cabbage leaves open on a clean work surface and divide mixture between the leaves. Fold the leaves around mixture and transfer to a lightly oiled ovenproof dish.

6. Pour tomato sauce over the stuffed leaves and bake at 425°F for 30 minutes.

BROWN LENTIL COTTAGE PIE

Serves 4.
8g fiber/330 calories per portion.

1 cup brown lentils
1 bay leaf
1 leek, sliced
2 carrots, sliced
1 onion, diced
1 teaspoon vegetable stock concentrate or 1 bouillon cube
1 tablespoon whole wheat flour
1 pound potatoes
2½ tablespoons unsalted butter
⅓ cup skimmed milk
1 free-range egg

1. Place the washed lentils in a saucepan with bay leaf. Cover with water and bring to the boil. Lower heat and simmer for 20 minutes.

2. Prepare the leek, carrots and onion and sauté in a frying pan with a smear of oil.

3. When the lentils are cooked remove bay leaf and drain, if necessary. Add the vegetables to the lentils and stock concentrate.

4. Stir in a few tablespoons boiling water. Sprinkle on the flour and stir well until mixture thickens.

5. Transfer mixture to an ovenproof dish.

6. Meanwhile scrub the potatoes and boil. When cooked, mash and cool.

7. Transfer the potatoes to a blender with the butter, milk and egg. Blend to smooth purée and spoon over the lentils.

8. Cover and bake at 400°F for 40 minutes.

RED LENTIL COTTAGE PIE

Serves 4.
10g fiber/350 calories per portion.

1 cup red lentils
1⅓ cups diced onion
1⅓ cups grated carrots
1 large green pepper
1 pound canned tomatoes
Sea salt
Freshly ground black pepper
2½ tablespoons unsalted butter or polyunsaturated margarine
2 tablespoons skimmed milk
2 cups potatoes, boiled and mashed

1. Pick over the lentils to remove any stones or grit. Wash well.

2. Place washed lentils in saucepan and cover with water. Bring to boil, lower heat and simmer for 20 minutes.

3. Put the lentils, onion, carrots, pepper and tomatoes in a saucepan and cook together for about 20 minutes. Break up the tomatoes with the back of a spoon to release their juice.

4. Mash fat and milk with potatoes. For smoother potatoes purée in a food processor after mashing.

5. Stir together lentils and vegetable mixture, season and place in an ovenproof dish. Top with mashed potatoes and broil to brown or reheat if necessary.

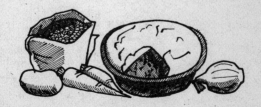

TOMATO SAUCE
Sauce contains 4g fiber and 55 calories.

1 pound tomatoes, chopped
²/₃ cup water
Bunch parsley tied with string
1 bay leaf
Sprig thyme
2 stalks celery, roughly chopped

1. Place all the ingredients in a heavy-based saucepan with well-fitting lid and simmer, covered, for 30 minutes.

2. Remove the bay leaf, thyme and parsley.

3. Place the rest of the ingredients in a blender and blend to a smooth sauce.

10

VEGETABLE SIDE DISHES

STUFFED TOMATOES
Serves 4.
5g fiber/150 calories each.

4 large beefsteak tomatoes
1 cup diced onion
1 clove garlic (optional)
1/2 cup peanuts, finely chopped
1 stalk celery, chopped
1 teaspoon Marmite
Few drops Tabasco
1/2 cup fresh whole wheat breadcrumbs

1. Slice tops from the tomatoes and using serrated-edged teaspoon remove seeds and pulp. Turn the tomatoes upside down to drain and place seeds and pulp in saucepan.

2. Add the onion, garlic, peanuts and celery to tomato pulp and cook over a low heat for 5 minutes.

3. Stir in the Marmite, Tabasco and breadcrumbs. Remove from heat and place the mixture in the tomatoes. Replace the tomato lids and hold in place with wooden cocktail picks.

4. Place the stuffed tomatoes in a lightly oiled ovenproof dish and bake at 350°F for 20 minutes.

BAKED ONIONS
Serves 4.
5½g fiber/190 calories per portion.

4 large onions
⅔ cup cooked brown rice
¾ cup roasted peanuts, chopped
1 medium-sized green pepper diced
Sea salt
Freshly ground black pepper
⅔ cup vegetable stock

1. Steam or boil the onions in their skins for 20 minutes. Drain and allow to cool slightly.

2. Mix the cooked rice with nuts and pepper and season to taste.

3. Slice the top and bottom from onion and press out the center of the onions, reserve. Place onions in an ovenproof dish.

4. Divide the rice mixture into 4 and fill the center of the onions.

5. Finely chop the reserved onion and mix with stock. Pour over the onions.

6. Cover and bake at 400°F for 30 minutes.

BRAISED RED CABBAGE
Serves 4.
9g fiber/80 calories per portion.

2 pounds red cabbage
1 pound cooking apples
1 tablespoon raw sugar
⅔ cup red wine vinegar
⅔ cup water

1. Shred the cabbage and wash well. Place in a large saucepan, or ovenproof dish with well-fitting lid.

2. Wash and grate or slice the apples, but do not peel. Add to the cabbage.

3. Add the sugar and pour over the vinegar and water.

4. Cook on top of the stove over gentle heat for 30 minutes or bake at 350°F for 40 minutes.

RATATOUILLE
Serves 4.
4g fiber/98 calories per portion.

1 tablespoon olive oil
1⅓ cups peeled and diced onion
2 cloves garlic, crushed
8 ounces eggplants, sliced
8 ounces zucchini, sliced
8 ounces green pepper, seeded and sliced
8 ounces tomatoes, skinned and chopped
2 tablespoons chopped parsley

1. Put the olive oil in a large heavy-based saucepan. Add the onion and garlic and sauté for 3 minutes.

2. Add the rest of the vegetables and stir together well. Cover and leave to simmer for about 40 minutes, stirring occasionally to prevent sticking.

3. Alternatively place mixture in an ovenproof dish with well-fitting lid and bake at 350°F for about 1 hour.

4. Before serving sprinkle with parsley and stir in.

SPINACH CHOUX BALLS

Makes 10.
4½g fiber/300 calories per ball.

2 cups water
½ cup unsalted butter or polyunsaturated margarine
2½ cups whole wheat flour
3 free-range egg yolks
½ teaspoon cayenne pepper

Filling:

½ cup unsalted butter or polyunsaturated margarine
1 cup whole wheat flour
2½ cups vegetable stock
1 cup frozen spinach or 2 cups fresh spinach
½ cup ricotta cheese

1. Place the water and fat in a saucepan and bring to boiling point.

2. Remove from heat and beat in the sieved flour.

3. Gradually beat in the egg yolks one at a time and the cayenne pepper until the mixture is smooth and shiny and leaves the sides of the pan in one lump.

4. Place pastry in a piping bag with ¾ in. plain nozzle and pipe 20 balls onto a lightly oiled baking tray.

5. Bake at 425°F for about 20 minutes, or until balls are golden brown and well risen and inserted skewer comes out clean.

6. To make the filling place butter and flour in saucepan over low heat and stir to make a *roux*.

7. Gradually add stock, stirring continuously to form a thick, smooth sauce.

8. Remove from heat and stir in finely chopped spinach. Cool.

9. Stir in the cheese and place in a piping bag with ¼ in. plain nozzle.

10. Insert nozzle into base of choux balls and fill with spinach mixture.

TURNIP PURÉE

Serves 4.
11g fiber/150 calories per portion.

2 pounds small turnips
1 pound carrots
Pinch sea salt
2½ tablespoons unsalted butter or polyunsaturated margarine
Freshly ground black pepper
2 tablespoons sour cream
Freshly chopped chervil to garnish

1. Scrub and dice the turnips, do not peel.

2. Scrub and dice the carrots, do not peel.

3. Place the turnips and carrots in a vegetable steamer or boil in the minimum of water until just cooked. Drain, reserving cooking liquid.

4. Add seasoning, butter, and sour cream and mash with a potato masher. For a finer purée place the mashed vegetables in a blender or food processor and blend.

5. Return to saucepan with a little of the reserved cooking liquid and reheat quickly before serving.

6. Garnish with chervil.

CARROT RUTABAGA PURÉE

Serves 4.
12g fiber/160 calories per portion.

2 pounds rutabaga
1 pound carrots
Sea salt
Freshly ground black pepper
2½ tablespoons unsalted butter or polyunsaturated margarine
2 tablespoons sour cream
Freshly chopped parsley to garnish

1. Scrub and dice the rutabaga, do not peel.

2. Scrub and dice the carrots, do not peel.

3. Place the rutabaga and carrots in a vegetable steamer or boil in minimum of water until just cooked. Drain, reserving cooking liquid.

4. Add seasoning, butter and sour cream and mash with potato masher. For finer purée place mashed vegetables in blender or food processor and blend.

5. Return to saucepan with a little of the reserved cooking liquid and reheat quickly before serving.

6. Garnish with parsley.

11.

DESSERTS

APRICOT RICE

Serves 4.
12½g fiber/380 calories per portion.

2 cups fresh or dried apricots, chopped
2½ tablespoons no-added-sugar apricot jam
¾ cup short grain brown rice
2½ cups skimmed milk
½ teaspoon nutmeg
Rind of 1 lemon
2½ tablespoons unsalted butter

1. Place the apricots in a saucepan and cover with boiling water. Cover and cook for about 10 minutes if fresh or 40 minutes if dried or until soft. Drain if necessary.

2. Stir jam into cooked apricots.

3. Place the rice in a saucepan with well-fitting lid and add milk, nutmeg, lemon rind and butter and simmer over low heat for about 40 minutes until the rice is cooked and the milk absorbed.

4. Pile the rice into the center of a serving dish and pour apricots over.

JACK HORNER CRUMBLE

Serves 4.
14g fiber/400 calories per portion.

2 cups prunes
8 ounces fresh plums
2 large cooking apples
1½ cups whole wheat flour
½ teaspoon mixed spice (clove, cinnamon, ginger, nutmeg)
⅓ cup polyunsaturated margarine
⅓ cup raw sugar

1. Pour boiling water over the prunes and soak overnight. Cook in boiling water for about 30 minutes, or until soft enough to remove pits.

2. Halve the plums and remove pits.

3. Core and thinly slice the unpeeled apples. Place in the saucepan with plums and heat gently for about 5 minutes, until juices run from the plums.

4. Lightly oil an ovenproof dish. Mix fruit together and place in dish. Add a couple of tablespoons of water.

5. Sieve the flour and spice into a separate bowl and add the fat.

6. Rub fat into flour until the mixture resembles breadcrumbs in texture.

7. Stir in the sugar and place on top of the fruit. Bake at 400°F for about 40 minutes.

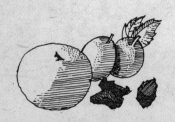

AUTUMN PUDDING

Serves 4.
18g fiber/300 calories per portion.

2 cups elderberries
2 cups blackberries
1 pound cooking apples
²/₃ cup water
1 small whole wheat loaf

1. Wash the elderberries and pull from stems. Place in a saucepan.

2. Wash and pick over the blackberries. Add to elderberries. Cover and cook over gentle heat for 10 minutes.

3. Core and slice the unpeeled apples and place in another saucepan with water. Cook until soft and beat to a pulp.

4. Line 1½ pint pudding mold with slices of bread trimmed to fit.

5. Mix together the fruits, reserving any juice and pour into the mold.

6. Place more bread on top of the fruit and pour over the reserved juice to soak bread thoroughly.

7. Place a saucer that fits inside the top of the mold in position and place weights on it to press it down. Leave overnight in fridge. Unmold before serving.

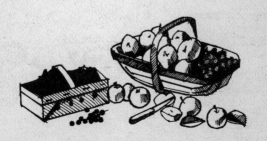

PRUNE JELLIES

Serves 4.
20g fiber/210 calories per portion.

4 cups prunes
1¼ cups red wine
⅔ cup water
1 orange
2 cups redcurrants
2 teaspoons gelatine or agar-agar

1. Place the prunes in a saucepan with the wine, water and rind of well-washed orange and bring to boil. Lower heat and simmer with lid on for 40 minutes or until prunes are cooked.

2. Trim the currants and place in another saucepan over a low heat. Cook for about 5 minutes. Remove and rub through sieve.

3. Soak the gelatine in the orange juice.

4. When the prunes are cooked strain the hot liquid onto gelatine, stirring all the time until the gelatine or agar-agar has dissolved.

5. Discard the orange rind and place prunes in bottom of 4 individual glass dishes.

6. Add the redcurrant juice to the prune juice and leave to cool. When on point of setting pour over prunes.

7. Place jellies in the fridge to cool before serving.

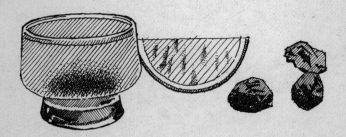

HOT FRUIT COMPOTE
Serves 4.
10g fiber/155 calories per portion.

2½ cups water
1 tablespoon clear honey
1 teaspoon cinnamon
1 teaspoon nutmeg
2 cloves
1 lemon
1 cup dried apricots
14 ounces peaches, canned in own juice or apple juice
⅔ cup golden seedless raisins

1. Place the water, honey, spices and juice and grated rind of well-washed lemon in a saucepan and bring to boil.

2. Add the apricots and reduce heat. Cover and simmer for 30 minutes.

3. Add the peaches and raisins and cook for further 10 minutes.

4. Serve hot. Offer natural yogurt separately.

Note: Any left-over compote is nice for breakfast on its own or with natural unsweetened yogurt.

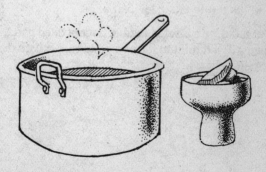

CHRISTMAS PUDDING

Serves 8.
6g fiber/450 calories per portion.

1⅓ cups raisins
½ cup blanched almonds, finely chopped
⅔ cup currants
⅔ cup golden seedless raisins
½ cup whole wheat flour
Pinch each of ground nutmeg, clove, ginger and cinnamon
1 cup whole wheat breadcrumbs
1 lemon, rind and juice
1 orange, rind and juice
2 cups unsalted butter or polyunsaturated margarine
2 tablespoons brandy
3 free-range eggs

1. Mix together all the dry ingredients.

2. Warm together in a saucepan the lemon juice, orange juice, butter and brandy. Remove from heat.

3. Beat the eggs well and add to the other liquids. Stir into dry ingredients.

4. Mixture should have a soft dropping consistency (drops easily from a raised spoon). If dry add more liquid, such as milk, water or juice.

5. Fill lightly oiled pudding mold with mixture, leaving about 1½ ins. at the top to allow for rising.

6. Cover mold with pleated double layer of oiled parchment paper topped with aluminum foil or a pudding cloth, tied beneath the rim with string.

7. Set mold in a large pan of boiling water or a steamer, or place in a pressure cooker.

8. Steam for 6 hours, adding boiling water as necessary. If using a pressure cooker steam according to manufacturer's instructions.

9. Allow to cool and store. Before serving on Christmas Day steam for a further 2 hours.

SUMMER PUDDING
Serves 4.
13g fiber/290 calories per portion.

2¹/₂ cups raspberries
2¹/₂ cups redcurrants
2¹/₂ cups blackcurrants
Small whole wheat loaf

1. Wash the fruit and trim currants.

2. Place fruit in a saucepan over a low heat. Cover and cook for 2 or 3 minutes only, until juices begin to run from the fruit.

3. Remove pan from heat and set aside.

4. Thinly slice the loaf, and line a pudding mold with the bread. Trim bread to fit.

5. Pour fruit and juice into the lined pudding mold and cover the fruit with more slices of bread.

6. Find a saucer that fits just inside the rim of the mold and place it on top of the bread and fruit.

7. Place a weight on top of the saucer and chill for several hours before inverting to remove from mold and serving.

PEACH GALETTE

Serves 4.
11g fiber/550 calories per portion.

2 cups dried peaches
½ cup unsalted butter, or polyunsaturated margarine
¾ cup oat bran and oat germ
¾ cup rolled oats
1 free-range egg
½ cup ricotta cheese

1. Place the dried peaches in a saucepan and cover with boiling water. Place lid on saucepan and simmer for about 30 minutes until soft. Drain and purée in blender.

2. Beat together half the purée (reserving half for filling) with the butter or margarine.

3. Add the oat bran and oat germ and rolled oats.

4. Beat in the egg.

5. Place the mixture in a piping bag with ¾ in. plain nozzle and pipe 3 rounds, each 6 in. in diameter, on lightly oiled baking tray.

6. Bake at 375°F for 25-30 minutes until firm to touch and golden brown. Remove from oven and cool.

7. Mix together remaining purée and ricotta.

8. Sandwich the 3 galette layers together with the dried peach and cheese purée.

RHUBARB FOOL
Serves 4.
7g fiber/215 calories per portion.

1 pound rhubarb, sliced into 1 in. pieces
1 tablespoon honey
1 teaspoon ground cinnamon
1 pound bananas
1¼ cups thick-set natural yogurt
½ cup wheat germ
½ cup chopped hazelnuts

1. Wash and slice the rhubarb. Place in a saucepan with honey, cinnamon and 6 tablespoons of water. Cover and cook over low heat for about 15 minutes.

2. Place the peeled and chopped bananas in a blender and blend to purée.

3. Add yogurt and mix thoroughly.

4. Add cooled rhubarb and mix again.

5. Turn into individual serving dishes.

6. Before serving top with wheat germ and nuts.

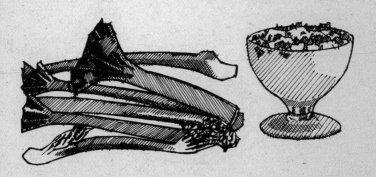

RHUBARB CRUMBLE

Serves 6.
5½g fiber/200 calories per portion.

1½ pounds rhubarb, sliced
1 tablespoon clear honey

Topping:

¾ cup whole wheat flour
¾ cup rolled oats
1 teaspoon ground cinnamon
⅓ cup polyunsaturated margarine
⅓ cup chopped dates

1. Wash and slice the rhubarb into 1 in. pieces.

2. Place in a saucepan with 2 tablespoons water and honey. Cover and cook over low heat for 5 minutes.

3. Transfer rhubarb to ovenproof dish.

4. Mix together the flour, oats and cinnamon.

5. Rub margarine into the flour mixture and stir in the dates.

6. Bake at 375°F for 40 minutes.

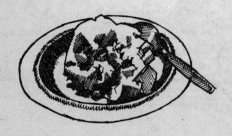

APRICOT AND COCONUT CRUMBLE

Serves 6.
18g fiber/300 calories per portion.

1 cup dried apricots
²/₃ cup raisins
¹/₃ cup golden seedless raisins
1 cup drained canned peach slices

Topping:

³/₄ cup whole wheat flour
³/₄ cup rolled oats
¹/₃ cup polyunsaturated margarine
²/₃ cup ground coconut
¹/₃ cup chopped dates

1. Place the apricots in a saucepan with boiling water and simmer for 40 minutes until soft. Cool and purée.

2. Stir in the golden seedless raisins and drained peaches. Place in an ovenproof dish and add a few tablespoons water.

3. Mix together the flour and oats.

4. Rub the margarine into the flour and oats and stir in the coconut and dates. Place on top of fruit.

5. Bake at 375°F for 30 minutes.

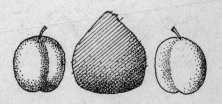

GOOSEBERRY CHEESECAKE

Serves 6.
4½g fiber/320 calories per portion.

1½ cups whole wheat flour
½ cup polyunsaturated margarine
Water to mix

Filling:

1 cup gooseberries
2 tablespoons clear honey
⅔ cup cottage cheese
1 free-range egg, separated
¼ cup ground almonds
¼ cup whole wheat semolina
1 free-range egg white
⅓ cup raisins, soaked in liqueur

1. Sieve the flour into a mixing bowl.

2. Rub fat into flour until the mixture resembles breadcrumbs in texture.

3. Form a soft dough by adding water.

4. Roll out on a lightly floured surface and carefully lift into base of a lightly oiled 8 in. cake tin or flan ring.

5. Trim the gooseberries and place in a saucepan with 2 tablespoons water. Cover and simmer for about 15 minutes. Cool and purée.

6. Beat together the honey, cheese, egg yolk, almonds and semolina.

7. Add the cooled gooseberries.

8. Whisk the egg white to firm peaks and quickly fold into mixture.

9. Place the raisins on the base of prepared pastry and pour over the gooseberry mixture.

10. Bake at 350°F for 40 minutes, or until set and firm to touch.

DE LUXE FRUIT SALAD

Serves 4.
4g fiber/105 calories per portion.

1 nectarine
1 dessert pear
1 peach
1 crisp eating apple with white flesh and red skin
1 banana
2 oranges
²⁄₃ cup orange juice
4 ounces green grapes

1. Wash all the fruit well.

2. Place orange juice in a serving dish and slice or dice all fruit straight into the juice to prevent browning. Do not peel fruit (except oranges and banana), but core if necessary, and remove seeds from grapes, if desired.

3. Reserve ¼ of each fruit for decoration.

4. Mix salad well.

5. To decorate, thinly slice each ¼ of fruit and arrange on top of the salad.

PASSION FRUIT SORBET

Serves 4.
4g fiber/140 calories per portion.

⅓ cup fructose (fruit sugar)
⅔ cup apple juice
9-10 passion fruits
Juice of ½ lemon
2 free-range egg whites

1. Place the fructose and apple juice in saucepan over low heat and dissolve fructose. Remove and cool.

2. Cut the fruits in half and scoop out pulp. Place in a bowl.

3. Add the lemon juice and fructose to pulp and pour mixture into a shallow tray or ice-cream maker and place in the freezer.

4. When the mixture is on point of setting remove and fold in stiffly beaten egg whites.

5. Place in a wetted and chilled container and return to freezer.

6. To serve use an ice-cream scoop to take sorbet from the container.

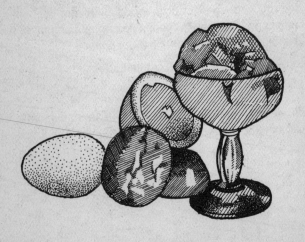

BLACKBERRY AND APPLE CRUMBLE

Serves 4.

8½g fiber/340 calories per portion.

1 pound cooking apples
1 lemon
8 ounces blackberries
½ cup whole wheat flour
½ cup rolled oats
½ cup unsalted butter or polyunsaturated margarine
⅓ cup finely chopped dates
¼ cup sunflower seeds

1. Core and slice the unpeeled apples and dress with lemon juice to prevent browning. Place in saucepan with the washed blackberries.

2. Place over low heat and cover. Cook for 5 minutes.

3. Turn the fruit into a lightly oiled ovenproof dish.

4. Mix together the flour and oats.

5. Rub fat into the flour mixture until it resembles breadcrumbs in texture.

6. Stir in dates and sunflower seeds and place the mixture on top of the fruit.

7. Bake at 375°F for 30 minutes.

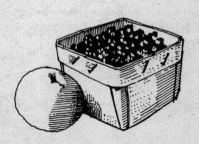

APRICOT GATEAU

Serves 6.
9g fiber/220 calories per portion.

3 free-range eggs
¼ cup clear honey
1 tablespoon boiling water
⅔ cup whole wheat flour

Topping:

1⅔ cups dried apricots
½ cup ricotta cheese
⅔ cup thick-set natural yogurt

1. Whisk the eggs and honey until pale in color and thick and ropey in texture.

2. Add water and quickly fold in the sieved whole wheat flour (and any bran left in the sieve) using a metal spoon.

3. Pour the mixture into a lightly oiled and lined 8 in. cake pan

4. Bake at 425°F for 15 minutes until golden brown and firm to the touch.

5. Remove from oven and leave in pan on rack to cool.

6. Cook the dried apricots in water until soft. Cool and purée.

7. Mix cold purée with cheese and yogurt.

8. Remove the cake from the tin, peel off paper. Using a long, sharp knife carefully slice cake into 3 layers. Sandwich together with apricot purée and cover top and sides of gateau with rest of mixture

12.

CAKES AND BAKES

HONEY AND HAZELNUT CAKE

Serves 4.
5g fiber/300 calories per portion.

4 free-range eggs, separated
²/₃ cup clear honey
1¹/₂ cups whole wheat flour
1 cup ground hazelnuts
¹/₃ cup skimmed milk

1. Whisk egg yolks and honey until light and thick in texture.

2. Fold in sieved flour and hazelnuts.

3. Stir in milk.

4. Whisk egg whites until they form stiff peaks.

5. Fold egg whites into mixture and pour into lightly oiled and lined 8 in. cake pan.

6. Bake at 350°F for 35-40 minutes or until golden brown and firm to touch.

CHRISTMAS CAKE

Serves 20, generously.
6g fiber/310 calories per portion.

2 cups whole wheat flour
1 teaspoon ground ginger
1 teaspoon ground nutmeg
1 teaspoon ground cinnamon
1 teaspoon ground cloves
1 cup ground almonds
2 cups currants
2 cups golden seedless raisins
2 cups raisins
1½ cups blanched almonds, finely chopped
2 cups unsalted butter
6 free-range eggs
1 orange
1 lemon
⅓ cup brandy (optional)

1. Sieve flour into mixing bowl with spices.

2. Stir in rest of dry ingredients.

3. In separate bowl cream butter and gradually add eggs. If mixture starts to separate add a little of the flour.

4. Stir butter and eggs into dry ingredients.

5. Scrub orange and lemon and grate rinds. Add the rinds and squeezed juice to the mixture.

6. If brandy is used stir it in.

7. Spoon mixture into 10 in. oiled and lined cake pan and bake for 1½ hours at 300°F, reduce heat to 250°F for a further 3 hours. Cover cake with brown or parchment paper or aluminum foil during the last 2 hours to prevent over-browning.

ROCK BUNS
Makes 12.
2g fiber/130 calories per bun.

2 cups whole wheat flour
2 teaspoons baking powder
1 teaspoon cinnamon
1/3 cup unsalted butter or polyunsaturated margarine
1/3 cup golden seedless raisins
1/3 cup currants
Grated rind of 1 lemon
1/3 cup milk
1 free-range egg

1. Sieve the flour, baking powder and spice into mixing bowl.

2. Rub fat into flour until the mixture resembles breadcrumbs in texture.

3. Stir in the golden seedless raisins, currants and lemon rind.

4. Stir milk into beaten egg and add to the dry ingredients to make them moist, but not sloppy.

5. Place a teaspoon of mixture into small, lightly oiled muffin tins or individual cake papers and roughen surface with a fork.

6. Bake at 400°F for 15 to 20 minutes.

Note: They are best eaten on the same day.

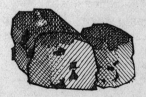

WHOLE WHEAT BREAD

Two loaves about 12 slices each.
1½-2g fiber/50-55 calories per slice.

4 cups whole wheat flour
Pinch sea salt
1¼ cups water at 98°F (37°C)
1½ tablespoons fresh yeast, or 1 tablespoon dried
1 vitamin C tablet, crushed
1 tablespoon corn oil
1 tablespoon molasses

1. Sieve flour and salt together into bowl.

2. Place water in bowl. The correct temperature can be achieved by using ⅓ boiling to ⅔ cold water.

3. Crumble yeast into water. Stir in crushed vitamin C tablet.

4. Add oil and molasses to yeast mixture and stir well.

5. Make a well in the center of the flour and pour in liquid. Stir well to form a firm dough.

6. Turn onto lightly floured work surface and knead for 10 minutes. Knead by stretching dough away from the body using the heel of the hand. When stretched lift furthest point of dough back over body of dough and press again, away from body.

7. After kneading return dough to bowl and cover to prevent drying out and crust forming. Leave to rest for 10 minutes.

8. Heat oven to 425°F and lightly oil two small loaf pans.

9. Return risen dough to work surface and knead again. Form into two sausage shapes three times the width of the pan and fold two ends under. Place in pans and cover with a teatowel again to prevent crust forming. Leave in warm place until doubled in size.

10. Glaze with milk or beaten egg and bake for 45 minutes. Bread is ready when it falls easily from pans and sounds hollow when tapped on the base.

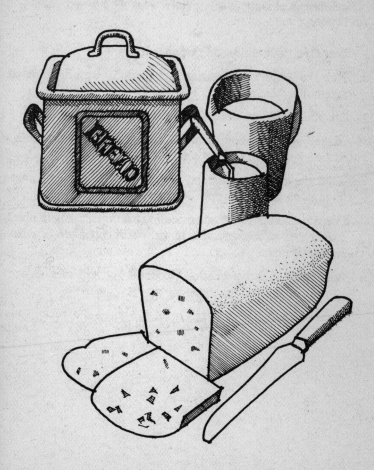

SULTANA SCONES

Makes one large round or 12 small scones.
23g fiber/1,160 calories, or
2g fiber/95 calories per scone.

2 cups whole wheat flour
1 teaspoon baking powder
¼ cup unsalted butter or polyunsaturated margarine
⅓ cup golden seedless raisins
⅔ cup buttermilk or skimmed milk with few drops of lemon juice added
Milk to glaze

1. Sieve the flour and baking powder into a bowl.

2. Rub the butter or margarine into the flour until the mixture resembles breadcrumbs in texture.

3. Stir the golden seedless raisins into mixture.

4. Make a well in the center of the dry ingredients and gradually add milk, stirring to form a soft dough.

5. Turn the dough onto a lightly floured board and gently knead for a couple of minutes until dough holds its shape and is pliable.

6. Form into a large round and place on a baking tray. Alternatively roll out to ¾ in. thickness and cut with pastry cutter into 12 wedge-shaped scones.

7. Glaze with milk and bake at 450°F for 10 to 15 minutes.

SPICED TEABREAD PLAIT
Makes about 12 slices.
4g fiber/150 calories per slice.

1 cup golden seedless raisins
1 cup raisins
1¼ cups apple juice
2 cups whole wheat flour
1 teaspoon mixed spice (clove, ginger, nutmeg)
½ teaspoon cinnamon
1 tablespoon fresh yeast
¼ cup unsalted butter or polyunsaturated margarine
Apple juice, warmed

1. Soak both raisins overnight in apple juice.

2. Sieve the flour and spices into a bowl and add bran from sieve.

3. Crumble yeast into flour.

4. Rub the margarine into the flour and yeast mixture.

5. Add the soaked fruit and warm juice to the flour mixture. Use only enough juice to make a firm dough.

6. Knead for 5 minutes on a floured surface. Return to bowl, cover and leave to rise.

7. When doubled in size punch down and knead again for 2 minutes. Divide the dough into three pieces and roll into sausage shapes. Press one end of the three pieces together and plait the dough.

8. Lift dough onto lightly oiled baking tray and glaze with milk or beaten egg. Bake at 400°F for 30-40 minutes — until a skewer comes out cleanly.

BROWN BREAD PUDDING

Serves 12.
4g fiber/150 calories per portion.

½ large whole wheat loaf, broken up roughly
¼ cup unsalted butter or polyunsaturated margarine
⅔ cup skimmed milk
2 tablespoons clear honey
2 free-range eggs, beaten
½ cup golden seedless raisins and raisins

1. Soak the bread in a little cold water or milk for at least 30 minutes.

2. Squeeze moisture from bread.

3. Melt fat in a saucepan with milk and add to the broken-up bread.

4. Stir in the honey and beaten eggs and beat to a soggy pulp.

5. Stir in the fruit and place in a lightly oiled cake or baking pan.

6. Bake for 1 hour at 350°F.

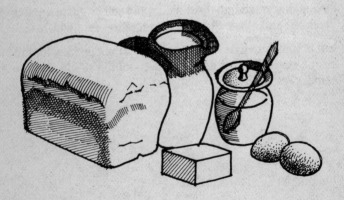

OATMEAL COOKIES

Makes 30 cookies.
1g fiber/52 calories per biscuit.

2 cups oatmeal
1¼ cups whole wheat flour
⅓ cup raw sugar
1 teaspoon baking powder
½ cup unsalted butter or polyunsaturated margarine
1 free-range egg
2 tablespoonsful skimmed milk

1. Mix together the oatmeal, flour, sugar and baking powder.

2. Rub in the fat to make a breadcrumb consistency.

3. Make a well in the center of the ingredients and add the beaten egg and milk. Mix to a stiff dough.

4. Lightly flour a work surface and roll dough out thinly. Cut into cookies with cutter.

5. Place cookies on a lightly oiled baking tray and brush with milk or beaten egg. Bake at 375°F for 15 minutes until golden brown.

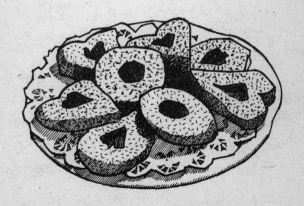

OATCAKES

Makes 20 oatcakes.
1g fiber/66 calories per oatcake.

2 cups oatmeal
½ cup whole wheat flour
1 teaspoon baking powder
5 tablespoons butter or polyunsaturated margarine
Boiling water to mix

1. Mix together the oatmeal, flour and baking powder.

2. Melt butter or margarine in a saucepan and stir into the dry ingredients.

3. Gradually add enough boiling water to make a dough, being careful not to add too much.

4. Knead lightly on a floured surface until the dough is firm enough to roll out.

5. Roll out and cut into triangles.

6. Slip a spatula under oatcakes and carefully lift onto a lightly oiled baking tray. Sprinkle with a little oatmeal and bake at 375°F for about 10-15 minutes.

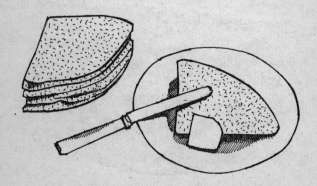

PRUNE DROPS

Makes about 20.
7g fiber/55 calories per drop.

¼ cup pitted prunes
¼ cup unsalted butter or polyunsaturated margarine
1 tablespoon clear honey
1 cup whole wheat flour
½ teaspoon baking powder
1 free-range egg
¼ cup slivered almonds

1. Wash the prunes and place in a saucepan. Cover with boiling water and cook until soft; about 40 minutes. Drain and cool before puréeing in blender.

2. Cream together the prune purée, margarine and honey.

3. Add the sieved flour and baking powder, returning bran from sieve to mixture.

4. Beat in the free-range egg.

5. Place mixture in a piping bag with a star nozzle and pipe small drops onto a lightly oiled baking tray.

6. Place an almond on top of each drop and bake at 400°F for 15 minutes.

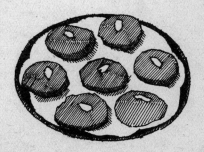

DATE AND PRUNE CAKE

Serves 8.
7g fiber/240 calories per portion.

½ cup unsalted butter or polyunsaturated margarine
¼ cup clear honey
2 free-range eggs, beaten
1½ cups whole wheat flour
2 teaspoons baking powder
1 teaspoon cinnamon
1 teaspoon mixed spice (clove, ginger, nutmeg)
1½ cups prunes, pitted and soaked overnight in apple juice
⅔ cup chopped dates
Water to mix

1. Beat the butter and honey together until light and fluffy.

2. Gradually add the eggs, beating continuously. If mixture shows signs of curdling add a little flour.

3. Sieve together the flour, baking powder and spices and fold into the butter.

4. Chop the soaked prunes and add prunes and dates to mixture.

5. Add water, if required, to form a soft mixture.

6. Turn mixture into a lightly oiled 8 in. cake pan and bake at 350°F for 1½ hours or until an inserted skewer comes out clean.

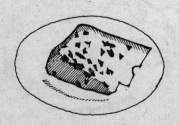

COCONUT CAKE

Serves 12.
3g fiber/190 calories per portion.

½ cup unsalted butter or polyunsaturated margarine
¼ cup clear honey
4 free-range eggs, separated
½ cup whole wheat flour
1 cup whole wheat semolina
1 teaspoon baking powder
1¼ cups ground coconut

1. Beat together the butter and honey until light and fluffy.

2. Gradually add egg yolks.

3. Sieve the flour, semolina and baking powder together and return bran from sieve to flour. Fold into the creamed mixture.

4. Stir in the coconut.

5. Whisk the egg whites until firm enough to hold stiff peaks. Fold into the mixture with a metal spoon.

6. Pour into a lightly oiled and lined cake pan and bake at 350°F for 40 minutes until golden brown and firm to the touch.

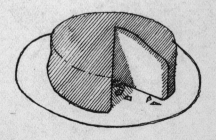

CINNAMON SWIRLS
Serves 4.
5g fiber/270 calories per portion.

1½ pounds sweet potato
2½ tablespoons unsalted butter or polyunsaturated margarine
⅓ cup sour cream
1 tablespoon honey
1 teaspoon ground cinnamon
1 free-range egg yolk, beaten
Grated rind of 1 orange
1 tablespoon skimmed milk

1. Scrub the potatoes and bake, unpeeled, at 400°F for 1 hour. Remove from oven, cut in half and scoop out all the flesh.

2. Pass flesh through a sieve or purée in a food processor and mix with fat, cream, honey, cinnamon and egg yolk.

3. Add grated rind of orange and turn the mixture into a piping bag with a ½ in. star nozzle.

4. Pipe rounds onto a lightly oiled baking tray and glaze with milk. Bake at 400°F for 20 minutes.

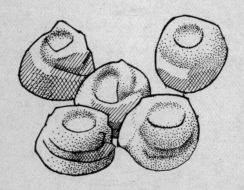

DATE FLAPJACKS

Makes 8.
3½g fiber/240 calories per flapjack.

½ cup polyunsaturated margarine
2½ tablespoons clear honey
2 cups rolled oats
⅔ cup chopped dates
⅓ cup water
1½ cups cooking apple, grated but not peeled

1. Melt the margarine and honey in a saucepan.

2. Stir in the oats. Set on one side.

3. Place the dates and water in another pan and cook to a soft pulp.

4. Add the apple to the dates and cook for a further few minutes.

5. Place half of the oat mixture in the bottom of a lightly oiled small cake pan.

6. Top with the date mixture and place the rest of the oats on the top. Level the mixture.

7. Bake at 350°F for 30 minutes, until golden brown.

8. Remove from the oven and mark into fingers. Do not remove from the pan until cold. Before removing re-cut sections.

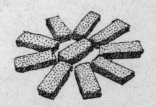

CARROT AND BANANA BREAD

Serves 8.
4g fiber/300 calories per portion.

2½ cups whole wheat flour
1 teaspoon baking powder
½ teaspoon mixed spice (clove, cinnamon, ginger, nutmeg)
½ cup unsalted butter or polyunsaturated margarine
⅔ cup dark brown sugar
2 free-range eggs
1 large banana, mashed
1 large carrot, grated
2 tablespoons sesame seeds

1.　Sieve the flour, baking powder and spice into a bowl.

2.　In another bowl cream the butter and sugar until light and fluffy.

3.　Beat the eggs and gradually add to the butter mixture.

4.　Stir in the banana, carrot and sesame seeds.

5.　Fold in the flour. Turn into a lightly oiled loaf pan and bake at 350°F for 45 minutes.

INDEX